Unraveling Social Justice Issues in Nursing

Naz Nami

Unraveling Social Justice Issues in Nursing

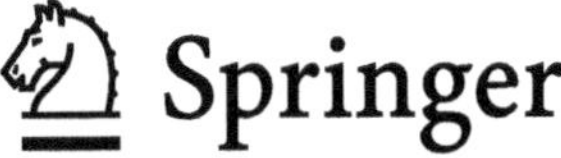

Springer

Naz Nami
University of Missouri–Kansas City (UMKC)
Kansas, MO, USA

ISBN 978-3-032-26511-1 ISBN 978-3-032-26512-8 (eBook)
https://doi.org/10.1007/978-3-032-26512-8

This Springer imprint is published by the registered company Springer Nature Switzerland AG
The registered company address is: Gewerbestrasse 11, 6330 Cham, Switzerland

This book is born from a journey of resilience of moving from surviving difficult experiences to finding purpose in serving others. Along the way, I have come to understand that healing, growth, and meaning are often shaped through connection.

I dedicate this work to my patients, whose strength, vulnerability, and humanity have taught me more than any textbook ever could. You have been my greatest teachers and the reason I strive to be a better clinician and a better person.

To my fellow nurses, who show up every day with compassion, courage, and quiet determination, this is for you. And to the future nurses who will carry this work forward, may you continue to challenge injustice and advocate for those whose voices are not always heard.

Most importantly, to my three beloved children, Izhak, Adam, and Isabel: you are my greatest source of love, purpose, and inspiration. Everything I do is for you.

With all my love.

Contents

About the Author

Naz Nami is a seasoned Psychiatric-Mental Health Nurse Practitioner (PMHNP) with more than a decade of clinical nursing experience and a dedicated advocate for neurodiversity, inclusion, and health equity. As an immigrant, lifelong learner, and autistic woman professional, she brings both lived experience and clinical expertise to her work, shaping a perspective grounded in resilience, authenticity, and person-centered care.

She began her academic journey at UC Berkeley before earning her nursing degree at Johns Hopkins University, where she developed a strong foundation in evidence-based practice and patient advocacy. She went on to complete her Psychiatric-Mental Health Nurse Practitioner degree at Boston College and is currently pursuing a PhD in Nursing Science. Her doctoral research focuses on developing inclusive and anti-ableist models of care that better support neurodivergent populations.

Deeply committed to justice and equity, Naz's work integrates clinical practice, research, and advocacy. Her identity as an autistic clinician informs her approach to care, emphasizing respect for diverse ways of thinking, communicating, and experiencing the world. Whether providing direct patient care, contributing to academic scholarship, or advocating for systemic change, she is dedicated to advancing healthcare systems that are accessible, equitable, and affirming for all individuals particularly those with neurodevelopmental and psychiatric differences.

Part I

Foundations of Social Justice in Nursing

1 Introduction to Social Justice in Nursing

Social justice has long been a guiding value in the profession of nursing, though its meaning has evolved in response to social change, healthcare inequities, and shifting cultural norms (Buettner-Schmidt and Lobo 2012; Reed and Rishel 2015). At its heart, social justice in nursing demands that all individuals, regardless of their race, gender, socioeconomic status, or ability, are afforded equal access to the conditions and resources necessary to achieve optimal health. This includes not only access to high-quality healthcare services but also the broader social determinants of health such as housing, education, employment, and safety. To embrace social justice is to commit to both advocacy and action, recognizing that health disparities are neither inevitable nor acceptable, but rather are the result of systemic inequities that nurses are ethically bound to challenge.

The American Nurses Association Code of Ethics makes explicit reference to social justice as a professional obligation. Provision 8, for instance, emphasizes the nurse's responsibility to advocate for human rights and to reduce health disparities, not only in the context of direct patient care but also within larger systems of healthcare and policy (American Nurses Association 2015). This ethical imperative reframes nursing as not only a caregiving profession but also a socially and politically engaged practice. Nurses are called to confront inequities both at the bedside and in society, highlighting the dual role of the nurse as both healer and advocate.

Understanding the concept of social justice within nursing requires situating it within a broader historical and philosophical framework. Social justice as a term has its origins in political philosophy, emphasizing fairness in the distribution of resources and opportunities (Rawls 1971; Fraser 1997). In healthcare, this translates to ensuring that no population is disproportionately burdened by disease or excluded from services due to structural barriers. Nursing, as a profession deeply intertwined with issues of vulnerability, illness, and care, is uniquely positioned to bring these principles into practice. Florence Nightingale's work during the Crimean War, for example, not only improved sanitary conditions and reduced mortality rates but also served as a form of social reform, drawing attention to the systemic neglect of

N. Nami, *Unraveling Social Justice Issues in Nursing*,
https://doi.org/10.1007/978-3-032-26512-8_1

soldiers' well-being. Later figures such as Lillian Wald, who founded the Henry Street Settlement in New York City, explicitly connected nursing with social justice by addressing poverty, immigrant health, and inadequate housing. These historical precedents establish a lineage of nursing as a vehicle for social change as much as a provider of medical care.

In contemporary contexts, the urgency of social justice in nursing is underscored by persistent health disparities across racial, socioeconomic, and geographic lines (World Health Organization 2020; Williams et al. 2019). Research consistently demonstrates that populations who experience systemic discrimination or economic marginalization face worse health outcomes, shorter life expectancies, and reduced access to preventive care. For example, Black Americans have higher rates of hypertension and maternal mortality compared to their white counterparts, outcomes that cannot be explained solely by genetics but are linked to social determinants of health and systemic racism within healthcare. Similarly, rural populations frequently encounter barriers related to geographic isolation, provider shortages, and lack of insurance coverage. These inequities demand not only clinical intervention but also structural advocacy, roles that nurses, given their close relationship with patients and communities, are particularly equipped to fulfill.

Social justice in nursing also encompasses the global context. The International Council of Nurses (2021) emphasizes that nurses worldwide are responsible for promoting equity, challenging unjust laws, and advocating for the health of vulnerable populations. This global vision recognizes that inequities are not confined to any one nation but are exacerbated by global forces such as poverty, climate change, conflict, and forced migration. Nurses working in resource-limited settings often confront stark disparities, where access to basic necessities such as clean water and vaccinations is unevenly distributed. Social justice thus requires a transnational commitment to solidarity and equity, positioning nursing as an advocate not just for individual patients but for global populations.

Equally important is the connection between social justice and health equity. While equality suggests treating everyone the same, equity requires acknowledging differences and tailoring interventions to meet specific needs (Braveman et al. 2017). For instance, providing equal access to flu vaccines may not achieve equitable outcomes if transportation barriers prevent rural populations from reaching clinics. In such cases, equity demands targeted interventions, such as mobile vaccination units or community-based outreach. Nurses, trained to consider the whole person and their environment, are particularly well-suited to identify these inequities and advocate for equitable solutions. Braveman, Arkin, Orleans, Proctor, and Plough emphasize that health equity is the practical manifestation of social justice in healthcare: it is what happens when systems actively work to eliminate avoidable and unfair disparities.

Understanding social justice in nursing also requires attention to power dynamics. Patients often enter healthcare systems in vulnerable positions, whether due to illness, lack of knowledge, or dependence on providers (Beauchamp and Childress 2019). Nurses, as frontline professionals, hold significant power in shaping patients' experiences of care. Exercising this power responsibly means ensuring that patients are respected, informed, and included in decision-making processes. It also means challenging institutional practices that perpetuate inequity, such as policies that restrict access based on ability to pay or protocols that fail to account for cultural differences. By addressing these power imbalances, nurses fulfill their ethical duty to promote justice not only at the bedside but also within healthcare institutions.

Finally, social justice in nursing is inseparable from advocacy. Advocacy involves more than speaking on behalf of patients; it also entails creating systems that amplify patients' own voices and empower communities to define their health priorities (Reed and Rishel 2015). For example, community health nurses may work alongside residents to design interventions that reflect cultural values and local needs, ensuring that solutions are not imposed but co-created. Advocacy also includes political engagement, as nurses lobby for legislation that expands healthcare coverage, funds public health programs, and addresses social determinants of health. In this way, social justice extends from the micro-level of nurse–patient interactions to the macro-level of policy and governance.

Historical Development of Social Justice in Nursing

The story of social justice in nursing cannot be told without situating the profession within its historical context (Stanhope and Lancaster 2020). Nursing emerged not only as a practice of caregiving but as a form of social reform, where the health of individuals was understood to be inextricably linked to the conditions of their environment. From the earliest pioneers of the profession to modern nursing leaders, advocacy for equity, fairness, and dignity has been at the core of nursing identity.

Florence Nightingale, often celebrated as the founder of modern nursing, demonstrated this connection between health and social conditions during the Crimean War (Stanhope and Lancaster 2020). Her reforms reduced mortality among soldiers not simply through medical treatment but through sanitary improvements, nutrition, and attention to environmental factors. Nightingale's vision extended beyond the battlefield, as she later advocated for public health reforms in England, emphasizing that poverty, overcrowding, and poor sanitation were as deadly as infectious diseases. In doing so, she laid the foundation for nursing as a profession deeply concerned with structural determinants of health, a theme that would echo throughout the profession's development.

In the early twentieth century, Lillian Wald advanced this vision through her work at the Henry Street Settlement in New York City (Stanhope and Lancaster 2020). Wald, often referred to as the founder of public health nursing, recognized that immigrant families living in poverty faced barriers not only to medical care but also to education, housing, and fair labor conditions. Her nurses provided bedside care, but they also engaged in advocacy, lobbying for better housing, safer workplaces, and public school nursing programs. Wald's integration of clinical practice with social reform remains one of the most powerful examples of nursing as a vehicle for social justice.

The legacy of Mary Eliza Mahoney further highlights the intersection of nursing with racial justice (Williams et al. 2019). As the first Black woman to become a professionally trained nurse in the United States, Mahoney entered a profession dominated by white women and often closed to people of color. Despite systemic racism, she not only excelled in her practice but also became a leading advocate for equity in nursing education and professional recognition. In 1908, she co-founded the National Association of Colored Graduate Nurses (NACGN), which provided a platform for Black nurses to organize against discrimination, promote professional excellence, and fight for inclusion in mainstream nursing organizations. Mahoney's contributions reflect how social justice has been a lived struggle within nursing itself, not only for patients but also for practitioners seeking equality within their own profession.

As the twentieth century progressed, nursing aligned itself with broader social movements (Reed and Rishel 2015). The civil rights era of the 1960s brought attention to the structural racism that shaped healthcare access and outcomes in the United States. Nurses participated in grassroots efforts to desegregate hospitals, expand access to care in underserved communities, and challenge discriminatory hiring practices within the profession. During the women's rights movement, nurses advocated for gender equity both in the workplace and in healthcare delivery, pressing for recognition of women's health issues and reproductive rights. These movements broadened the scope of nursing advocacy, embedding the principles of social justice within the fight for human rights more broadly.

Globally, nursing has also played a central role in advancing equity and justice (International Council of Nurses 2021). In low- and middle-income countries, nurses often serve as the backbone of healthcare systems, providing essential care in contexts of scarcity. Figures such as Sister Elizabeth Kenny, who pioneered innovative treatments for polio in Australia, demonstrate how nurses have historically pushed against the boundaries of established medicine to advocate for better patient outcomes. Internationally, organizations such as the International Council of Nurses (ICN) have positioned social justice as a global mandate, calling on nurses to address disparities in access to vaccines, clean water, maternal health, and primary care. The recognition that health is a universal human right has long connected nursing to movements for global equity.

By the end of the twentieth century, social justice was no longer just implicit in nursing practice but explicitly codified in professional ethics (American Nurses Association 2015; International Council of Nurses 2021). The American Nurses Association and the ICN both embedded social justice into their codes of ethics, framing it as a non-negotiable component of professional identity. Nurses were called not only to care for individuals but to act as advocates for communities, policymakers, and systems. The expectation shifted from individual discretion to collective responsibility, affirming that social justice is a shared mandate of the profession.

Today, this historical legacy informs the ways nurses approach twenty-first-century challenges such as systemic racism, health disparities, climate change, and global pandemics (Williams et al. 2019; World Health Organization 2020). Each of these crises reveals inequities in access to resources, treatment, and outcomes, making the role of nurses as advocates for justice more critical than ever. Just as Nightingale responded to the unsanitary conditions of military hospitals, or Wald to the poverty of immigrant communities, nurses today must respond to inequities laid bare by COVID-19, structural racism, and widening gaps in access to care. The history of nursing demonstrates that the profession is most powerful when it marries the science of care with the pursuit of justice.

Ethical Foundations, Barriers, and Contemporary Challenges

Nursing's connection to social justice is not incidental; it is deeply rooted in the ethical frameworks that guide the profession (American Nurses Association 2015; Reed and Rishel 2015). Ethics serve as the compass for nursing practice, directing how nurses engage with patients, families, colleagues, and communities. Beyond clinical competence, nurses are called to integrate values of fairness, dignity, and advocacy into their everyday practice. This ethical imperative is what transforms nursing from a purely technical profession into one that is profoundly moral and socially engaged.

The American Nurses Association's (ANA) Code of Ethics establishes social justice as a central principle. Provision 8, which calls on nurses to "reduce health disparities and advocate for human rights," expands the scope of nursing ethics beyond individual patient encounters and into the realm of communities, policies, and systems (ANA 2015). Similarly, the International Council of Nurses Code of Ethics emphasizes nurses' responsibility to promote equity and to challenge unjust structures in their societies. By embedding justice within their ethical codes, both organizations affirm that nurses cannot remain neutral in the face of inequity.

Philosophical frameworks in biomedical ethics also illuminate the importance of justice in healthcare. Beauchamp and Childress (2019), in their widely used model, identify justice as one of the four principles of biomedical ethics, alongside autonomy, beneficence, and non-maleficence. For nurses, justice demands more than fairness in the distribution of resources; it also requires active resistance to systems that exploit or neglect vulnerable populations. This principle places the burden of advocacy directly onto healthcare professionals, obligating them to identify inequities and to intervene where possible. Despite this clear ethical mandate, numerous barriers impede the integration of social justice into nursing practice. These barriers exist at multiple levels: structural, institutional, and personal.

At the structural level, healthcare systems themselves are often designed in ways that reproduce inequities (Braveman et al. 2017; World Health Organization 2020). In the United States, a reliance on employer-based insurance leaves millions uninsured or underinsured, disproportionately affecting racial minorities and low-income individuals. Nurses who care for these populations frequently witness the consequences of systemic exclusion patients who delay care due to costs, families forced to choose between paying rent and purchasing medications, or rural communities without access to specialized services. Structural inequities also manifest globally, where the uneven distribution of resources leaves entire regions without adequate healthcare infrastructure.

At the institutional level, inequities can be reinforced through policies, procedures, and workplace cultures (Reed and Rishel 2015). Hospitals may lack diversity in leadership, perpetuating decision-making that fails to reflect the needs of marginalized communities. Implicit bias in clinical decision-making may result in minority patients receiving less pain medication or fewer referrals for specialty care compared to white patients with similar conditions. Institutions may also fail to provide adequate interpreter services, leaving patients with limited English proficiency at risk of misdiagnosis or poor adherence to treatment plans.

At the personal level, nurses themselves may carry unconscious biases shaped by broader societal prejudices (Beauchamp and Childress 2019; Williams et al. 2019). These biases can subtly influence how nurses interpret patient behavior, communicate with families, or prioritize care. While few nurses intend to discriminate, unchecked biases can nonetheless contribute to disparities in health outcomes. The recognition of personal bias, therefore, is a critical step toward practicing ethically in a multicultural and diverse society.

Contemporary examples illustrate both the challenges and the possibilities of practicing social justice in nursing. Consider the case of maternal health disparities in the United States, where Black women face significantly higher rates of maternal mortality than white women (Williams et al. 2019). Nurses working in maternity care settings have begun to respond by advocating for culturally competent prenatal programs, pushing for policies that address social determinants of health such as housing and nutrition, and implementing listening sessions to ensure that women's voices are centered in their care. These efforts represent the translation of ethical commitments into practical interventions.

Another example can be seen in psychiatric nursing, where stigma and discrimination against individuals with mental illness often result in inadequate treatment (Reed and Rishel 2015). Nurses in these settings have worked to develop trauma-informed care models that recognize the impact of systemic oppression, poverty, and racism on mental health. By reframing patients' struggles within a broader social context, nurses not only provide more compassionate care but also advocate for systemic reforms in mental health policy and funding.

Globally, nurses have taken leading roles in addressing health inequities exacerbated by crises such as the COVID-19 pandemic (International Council of Nurses 2021; World Health Organization 2020). In many low- and middle-income countries, nurses were the primary healthcare providers during the pandemic, often operating with limited protective equipment and resources. Their advocacy for equitable vaccine distribution, public health education, and stronger health infrastructure exemplifies social justice in practice at the global scale. These actions reflect both the resilience of the nursing workforce and the ethical imperative to confront inequities in times of crisis.

Taken together, the ethical frameworks of nursing and biomedical ethics provide clear direction for integrating social justice into practice (American Nurses Association 2015; Beauchamp and Childress 2019). However, the persistence of structural, institutional, and personal barriers demonstrates that achieving justice is not automatic. It requires deliberate effort, continuous reflection, and systemic reform. Nurses must remain vigilant against complacency, recognizing that the ethical duty to advocate for equity extends across all levels of practice from bedside care to boardrooms, from local communities to global policy forums.

Education, Research, and Leadership for Social Justice

Education is one of the most powerful tools for embedding social justice within the profession of nursing (Reed and Rishel 2015). From the earliest stages of training, nursing students are not only taught clinical skills but are also introduced to the ethical foundations of care. Increasingly, nursing schools are integrating social justice into curricula, ensuring that future nurses understand health not only as a biological outcome but also as a social phenomenon shaped by inequality, discrimination, and access to resources.

In academic settings, the inclusion of cultural competence and cultural humility has become a cornerstone of nursing education (Campinha-Bacote 2011). Cultural competence refers to the ability of nurses to understand and respect the cultural backgrounds of patients, while cultural humility emphasizes an ongoing process of self-reflection and learning, recognizing that no clinician can master every culture but must instead remain open and responsive. These concepts align directly with social justice, as they prepare nurses to care equitably for diverse populations and to avoid imposing assumptions or stereotypes in clinical practice.

Beyond cultural competence, nursing schools are incorporating social determinants of health into training (World Health Organization 2020; Braveman et al. 2017). Students learn how poverty, education, housing, employment, and systemic discrimination influence health outcomes. By recognizing these factors, nurses are better equipped to identify inequities in practice and to advocate for systemic solutions. For example, a nurse who understands the relationship between housing instability and chronic illness may be more likely to advocate for social services referrals or to collaborate with community organizations. Integrating these concepts into nursing curricula ensures that graduates view their role not narrowly as clinical caregivers but broadly as advocates for health equity.

Clinical placements and community-based experiences also play an important role in shaping nurses' commitment to social justice (Stanhope and Lancaster 2020). Students who work in underserved neighborhoods, rural clinics, or international service-learning programs gain firsthand experience of health disparities. These experiences often serve as transformative moments, highlighting the structural inequities that shape health outcomes. Faculty can enhance these experiences by encouraging reflection, dialogue, and critical analysis, helping students connect individual patient stories to broader systemic patterns of injustice.

Nursing education also prepares future nurses to become leaders and change agents (Reed and Rishel 2015). Courses in health policy, ethics, and leadership increasingly emphasize the role of nurses in shaping healthcare systems and advocating for reform. Graduates are encouraged not only to provide care but also to engage in professional organizations, influence legislation, and contribute to policy discussions. In this way, nursing education serves as the foundation for a nursing workforce capable of addressing both clinical and systemic inequities.

Alongside education, nursing research and evidence-based practice are essential for advancing social justice in nursing (Reed and Rishel 2015). Evidence provides the foundation for advocacy, enabling nurses to highlight inequities with data and to propose solutions grounded in research. For example, epidemiological studies documenting racial disparities in maternal mortality have fueled advocacy efforts to expand Medicaid coverage, increase funding for community-based maternity programs, and improve cultural competence training for providers. Similarly, research demonstrating inequities in pain management across racial groups has led to calls for bias training and reforms in clinical decision-making tools.

Nurses have contributed to this body of research in large (Reed and Rishel 2015). As nursing scholars, they investigate the experiences of marginalized populations, evaluate the effectiveness of interventions, and develop models of care that promote equity. Participatory nursing action research, in which communities are actively involved in shaping research questions and interventions, has become an increasingly important approach in nursing scholarship. This methodology reflects the principles of social justice by empowering communities to define their own priorities and by ensuring that research outcomes directly benefit those who are most affected.

Leadership is another critical dimension of nursing's commitment to social justice (American Nurses Association 2015; Reed and Rishel 2015). Nurses occupy leadership roles in hospitals, public health agencies, academic institutions, and professional organizations. In these positions, they have the opportunity to influence policy, resource allocation, and organizational culture. Nurse leaders who prioritize equity can ensure that institutional policies promote diversity, address bias, and allocate resources to underserved populations. For example, a nurse leader in a hospital setting might advocate for the establishment of interpreter services, recognizing that language barriers compromise both equity and patient safety.

At the policy level, nurses are increasingly recognized as key stakeholders in legislative advocacy (American Nurses Association 2015). Organizations such as the American Nurses Association and the National League for Nursing actively lobby for policies that expand access to care, address social determinants of health, and promote workforce diversity. Individual nurses also contribute by meeting with legislators, providing testimony at hearings, and participating in grassroots advocacy campaigns. By leveraging their expertise and their trusted status in society, nurses can shape policies that advance social justice on a broad scale.

Finally, leadership in social justice requires addressing inequities within the profession itself (Stanhope and Lancaster 2020). Nursing has historically struggled with issues of diversity and inclusion, with people of color, men, and individuals from lower socioeconomic backgrounds underrepresented in the workforce. Efforts to diversify nursing education and leadership are essential not only for equity within the profession but also for improving patient care, as research demonstrates that diverse teams provide more innovative and effective solutions. By fostering diversity within their own ranks, nurses model the values of equity and justice that they advocate for in society.

Taken together, education, research, and leadership form a powerful triad for advancing social justice in nursing (Reed and Rishel 2015). Education equips nurses with the knowledge, skills, and ethical frameworks needed to recognize inequities. Research provides the evidence base for advocacy and reform. Leadership ensures that nurses have a seat at the table where decisions are made, enabling them to influence policies and systems. Together, these elements ensure that nursing remains not only a profession of caregiving but also a profession of advocacy, committed to dismantling inequities and advancing health equity for all.

Case Studies, Global Perspectives, and a Call to Action

To fully appreciate the significance of social justice in nursing, it is useful to examine concrete examples of how these principles are applied in practice (Reed and Rishel 2015). Case studies provide a window into the lived realities of inequities and demonstrate how nurses respond to injustice at both individual and systemic levels.

One particularly striking example is found in maternal health. In the United States, Black women are three to four times more likely to die from pregnancy-related causes than white women (Williams et al. 2019). This disparity cannot be explained by socioeconomic status alone, as even well-educated and insured Black women face higher risks. Nurses working in maternity care have been at the forefront of responding to this crisis. By advocating for culturally competent care, improving communication between providers and patients, and lobbying for expanded prenatal and postpartum support services, nurses translate the abstract principle of social justice into tangible interventions. Some hospitals have established nurse-led listening programs that ensure Black women's voices are heard during pregnancy and childbirth, reducing the likelihood that symptoms will be dismissed or ignored. These initiatives highlight the essential role of nurses in addressing inequities that stem from racism and bias within the healthcare system.

Another case study can be found in the treatment of individuals with mental illness. Historically, patients with psychiatric diagnoses have faced stigma, neglect, and even abuse within healthcare systems (Reed and Rishel 2015). Nurses practicing within psychiatric and mental health settings have advanced social justice by promoting trauma-informed care, which recognizes that many mental health struggles are rooted in systemic oppression, poverty, and violence. For instance, community psychiatric nurses have collaborated with housing organizations to address homelessness among individuals with chronic mental illness. By acknowledging that secure housing is as important to recovery as medication or therapy, these nurses exemplify a justice-oriented approach that addresses the root causes of poor health outcomes.

Case studies also emerge in global health contexts. During the COVID-19 pandemic, inequities in vaccine distribution revealed the deep divide between wealthy and low-income nations (World Health Organization 2020). While countries in the Global North secured large supplies of vaccines, many low-income countries struggled to access even minimal doses. Nurses across the world played crucial roles in advocating for equitable distribution, participating in community education campaigns to combat vaccine misinformation, and ensuring that vulnerable populations were prioritized once vaccines became available. In rural African villages, for example, nurse-led mobile clinics brought vaccines to populations who otherwise would have been excluded from protection. These efforts illustrate nursing's global responsibility to promote justice in times of crisis.

Looking more broadly, global perspectives demonstrate that social justice in nursing takes different forms depending on cultural, political, and economic contexts (World Health Organization 2020). In some countries, nurses fight for the most basic resources such as clean water, sanitation, and access to antibiotics, while in others, they challenge subtle but pervasive inequities in high-tech healthcare systems. For example, in Canada and Australia, Indigenous populations face profound health disparities rooted in historical injustices and ongoing marginalization. Nurses working in Indigenous communities advocate for culturally safe care that respects traditional healing practices and addresses the intergenerational trauma caused by colonization. In the United Kingdom, nurses have played prominent roles in campaigns to preserve universal healthcare access under the National Health Service, recognizing that cuts to public funding disproportionately harm the most vulnerable populations. These examples illustrate that while the manifestations of injustice differ, the nursing response is unified by a commitment to equity and dignity.

The global perspective also highlights the interconnectedness of health and justice. Climate change, for example, disproportionately affects communities already marginalized by poverty, race, or geography (World Health Organization 2020). Nurses are increasingly called upon to advocate for climate justice, recognizing that rising temperatures, extreme weather events, and pollution exacerbate health disparities. Similarly, global migration and refugee crises present challenges to health systems, demanding responses that combine clinical care with advocacy for human rights. Nurses at refugee camps in Jordan, for instance, not only provide essential medical services but also advocate for policies that ensure access to education, housing, and legal protection. Such efforts reinforce the understanding that social justice in nursing transcends borders and requires solidarity on a global scale.

As this chapter has demonstrated, social justice is not a peripheral concept in nursing but rather a core ethical and professional obligation (American Nurses Association 2015; Reed and Rishel 2015). From the historical legacies of Florence Nightingale, Lillian Wald, and Mary Eliza Mahoney to the modern struggles against systemic racism, maternal mortality, and global inequities, nursing has consistently been positioned as both a clinical and a social force. The principles of equity, dignity, and advocacy run through the very fabric of the profession, shaping its practices, its education, and its codes of ethics.

The path forward, however, is not without challenges for nurses. Structural, institutional, and personal barriers continue to impede the realization of justice in healthcare (Braveman et al. 2017; Williams et al. 2019). Profit-driven healthcare systems, discriminatory practices, implicit bias, and underrepresentation in leadership all conspire to maintain inequities. Overcoming these obstacles requires sustained commitment, systemic reform, and personal reflection. Nurses must not only advocate for their patients but also examine their own practices, assumptions, and roles within unjust systems.

Yet the opportunities are profound. Nurses represent the largest segment of the healthcare workforce worldwide and consistently rank as the most trusted professionals in public opinion surveys (International Council of Nurses 2021). This trust, coupled with their intimate proximity to patients and communities, places nurses in a unique position to lead social justice initiatives. Whether through policy advocacy, research, leadership, or bedside care, nurses have the capacity to transform healthcare systems into engines of equity rather than vehicles of exclusion.

The call to action is clear: nurses must continue to embrace their role as advocates for social justice (American Nurses Association 2015; International Council of Nurses 2021). This involves acknowledging inequities, supporting systemic change, and committing to lifelong learning and reflection. It means engaging in legislative advocacy, partnering with communities, and amplifying the voices of those most affected by inequity. It requires building solidarity across borders and recognizing that justice in healthcare is inseparable from justice in society as a whole.

As we conclude this chapter, it is worth remembering that the pursuit of social justice is not an optional component of nursing practice; it is its very essence (Reed and Rishel 2015). To care for patients is to care about the conditions that shape their health. To heal is to challenge the systems that cause harm. As a nurse, to advocate is to fulfill the deepest ethical commitments of the profession. Social justice, then, is not simply part of what it means to be a nurse: it is what defines nursing at its most authentic, its most ethical, and its most transformative.

References

American Nurses Association. Code of ethics for nurses with interpretive statements. American Nurses Association; 2015.

Beauchamp TL, Childress JF. Principles of biomedical ethics. 8th ed. Oxford University Press; 2019.

Braveman P, Arkin E, Orleans T, Proctor D, Plough A. What is health equity? And what difference does a definition make? Robert Wood Johnson Foundation; 2017.

Buettner-Schmidt K, Lobo ML. Social justice: a concept analysis. J Adv Nurs. 2012;68(4):948–58. https://doi.org/10.1111/j.1365-2648.2011.05856.x.

Campinha-Bacote J. Delivering patient-centered care in the midst of a cultural conflict: the role of cultural competence. Online J Issues Nurs. 2011;16(2):1–8. https://doi.org/10.3912/OJIN.Vol16No02Man05.

Fraser N. Justice interruptus: critical reflections on the "postsocialist" condition. Routledge; 1997.

International Council of Nurses. Code of ethics for nurses. International Council of Nurses; 2021. https://www.icn.ch/nursing-policy/icn-code-ethics.

Rawls J. A theory of justice. Harvard University Press; 1971.

Reed S, Rishel CJ. Nursing ethics and social justice: foundations and education. J Nurs Educ. 2015;54(Suppl. 6S):S39–43. https://doi.org/10.3928/01484834-20150518-10.

Stanhope M, Lancaster J. Public health nursing: population-centered health care in the community. 10th ed. Elsevier; 2020.

Williams DR, Lawrence JA, Davis BA. Racism and health: evidence and needed research. Annu Rev Public Health. 2019;40(1):105–25. https://doi.org/10.1146/annurev-publhealth-040218-043750.

World Health Organization. Social determinants of health. 2020. https://www.who.int/health-topics/social-determinants-of-health.

2 Ableism and Disability Rights in Nursing

Introduction to Ableism in Nursing

The nursing profession has long been grounded in principles of compassion, advocacy, and respect for human dignity (American Nurses Association 2015). These values are central to both its practice and its ethical commitments. Yet, despite these guiding ideals, nursing, like the rest of healthcare, exists within a broader social framework that has historically marginalized and excluded certain populations. Among the most enduring and insidious forms of marginalization is ableism, a system of discrimination and oppression directed toward people with disabilities. Although less frequently discussed than racism or sexism in healthcare, ableism profoundly shapes the experiences of patients, families, and healthcare providers.

Ableism is more than individual prejudice or bias (Nami 2025; Buettner-Schmidt and Lobo 2012). It is a deeply entrenched system of beliefs, practices, and structures that privilege those considered "able-bodied" or "neurotypical" while devaluing those whose bodies or minds fall outside socially accepted norms. It manifests in assumptions that disabled lives are less valuable, in practices that restrict access to care, and in policies that fail to account for the needs of disabled people. For nurses whose daily work requires close interactions with patients across diverse backgrounds understanding and addressing ableism is not optional but fundamental to ethical practice.

In healthcare, ableism often goes unrecognized because it is embedded in "common sense" assumptions about health, independence, and quality of life (Nami 2025; Shakespeare 2013). For instance, the frequent emphasis on "restoring function" or "returning to normal" positions disability as a negative deviation rather than a natural variation of human existence. Nursing, which prides itself on holistic care, may inadvertently reinforce ableist attitudes when patients' capacities and strengths are overlooked in favor of focusing solely on deficits. Recognizing these patterns is the first step toward dismantling them.

N. Nami, *Unraveling Social Justice Issues in Nursing*,
https://doi.org/10.1007/978-3-032-26512-8_2

A draft of my working paper (Nami 2025) on ableism provides a structured foundation for exploring how this form of discrimination operates in nursing. Using Walker and Avant's method of concept analysis, this draft describes ableism in terms of its defining attributes (e.g., privileging able-bodied norms, stigmatizing difference), antecedents (e.g., cultural ideals of productivity, the medicalization of disability), and consequences (e.g., exclusion, psychological harm, health disparities). Importantly, this analysis underscores that ableism is not limited to overt acts of discrimination. It also includes subtle and structural forms of bias that permeate healthcare delivery. Nurses may perpetuate ableism unintentionally through diagnostic overshadowing attributing unrelated symptoms to a patient's disability or by neglecting to provide accessible communication for individuals with sensory or cognitive impairments.

Understanding ableism in nursing also requires situating it within broader historical and theoretical contexts (Oliver 1990; Shakespeare 2013). Historically, disabled people were primarily understood through the medical model of disability, which frames disability as an individual pathology to be treated or corrected. This model dominated healthcare for centuries, shaping everything from clinical practices to public health policy. While it contributed to advances in rehabilitation and treatment, it also perpetuated the belief that disabled bodies are inherently deficient.

In contrast, the social model of disability, developed through disability rights movements in the twentieth century, shifted the focus away from impairments and toward societal barriers (Oliver 1990; Charlton 1998). According to this perspective, disability arises not from the body or mind itself but from inaccessible environments, discriminatory attitudes, and exclusionary systems. For example, a person who uses a wheelchair is only "disabled" when public spaces lack ramps or elevators. This paradigm was crucial in reshaping understandings of disability and advancing protections such as the Americans with Disabilities Act (ADA).

For nurses, adopting the social model provides a justice-oriented framework for practice (Oliver 1990; American Nurses Association 2015). It invites us to ask not only "what is wrong with this patient?" but also "what barriers in the environment, systems, or attitudes are preventing this patient from achieving optimal health?" This shift aligns with holistic care and with the principles of social justice articulated in the ANA Code of Ethics.

Ableism rarely operates alone. It intersects with other systems of oppression, including racism, sexism, and classism (Charlton 1998; Garland-Thomson 2017). Disabled people of color, for example, face compounded disadvantages as they encounter both racial and ableist discrimination in healthcare. Women with disabilities may be denied reproductive autonomy due to paternalistic attitudes. Low-income individuals with disabilities often face systemic barriers to insurance, accessible housing, and employment. These realities emphasize the need for an intersectional framework in nursing practice, one that recognizes the ways in which different forms of discrimination converge.

The consequences of ableism in healthcare are profound. Disabled individuals experience higher rates of unmet health needs, poorer health outcomes, and reduced life expectancy compared to nondisabled peers (Buettner-Schmidt and Lobo 2012; World Health Organization 2011). These inequities are not inevitable but result from structural exclusion and discriminatory practices. For example, disabled patients are less likely to receive preventive screenings not due to clinical contraindications but because facilities are inaccessible or providers assume such care is unnecessary. Similarly, disabled individuals often report being dismissed or disbelieved by healthcare professionals, leading to delays in diagnosis and treatment. Such disparities undermine both ethical principles of justice and the core nursing values of respect and advocacy.

Addressing ableism requires action at multiple levels (Nami 2025; World Health Organization 2011). Education must prepare students to recognize and challenge ableism, incorporating disability studies perspectives and cultural humility into training. Research should examine how ableism shapes health outcomes and guide inclusive interventions. At the policy level, nurses can advocate for reforms that advance accessibility, equity, and inclusion, ensuring that disabled voices are integral to decision-making.

This chapter will explore ableism and disability rights in nursing more deeply, using the draft of my paper as a foundation while expanding into historical, theoretical, and practice-based contexts (Nami 2025). It will move from definitions and frameworks to real-world examples of ableism in practice, before turning to strategies for developing an anti-ableist nursing profession. The goal is to demonstrate that dismantling ableism is not simply a matter of individual goodwill but requires systemic change in education, practice, and policy.

By the end of this chapter, it will be clear that addressing ableism is not peripheral to nursing but central to its mission (American Nurses Association 2015; Nami 2025). Advocating for human dignity, promoting equity, and delivering holistic care all require a firm commitment to disability justice. Nurses must recognize that disabled people are not passive recipients of care but active participants whose lived experiences bring essential expertise. Only by embracing this perspective can nursing fulfill its ethical obligations and contribute to a more inclusive and equitable healthcare system.

Historical and Theoretical Foundations of Ableism in Nursing

The persistence of ableism in nursing and healthcare cannot be fully understood without tracing its historical roots and theoretical underpinnings (Oliver 1990; Barnes and Mercer 2010). The way societies have defined, classified, and responded to disability has always been shaped by prevailing cultural, medical, and political contexts. For centuries, disabled bodies and minds have been subject to stigma, exclusion, and paternalism, with healthcare often reinforcing rather than dismantling these inequities. By examining the historical development of disability perspectives and the theoretical models that have shaped nursing practice, it becomes clear why ableism is so deeply embedded in healthcare and why systemic change is necessary.

The Medical Model of Disability

For much of modern history, disability was defined and addressed through the medical model of disability, which frames disability primarily as an individual pathology or defect to be treated, rehabilitated, or cured (Oliver 1990; Shakespeare 2013). Rooted in the nineteenth-century scientific medicine, this model positioned disabled people as patients whose bodies or minds deviated from the "normal" standard of health. The focus was on correction and normalization: physicians and nurses aimed to restore patients to "wholeness" by eliminating or mitigating impairments.

The medical model contributed to important advances in rehabilitation, prosthetics, and treatment of chronic illness (Barnes and Mercer 2010). However, it also fostered problematic assumptions. It encouraged healthcare workers to view disability as a problem located solely in the individual, while ignoring the role of societal barriers. Under this model, the success of nursing care was often judged by whether a patient could return to "normal function," sidelining those whose impairments were permanent. Disabled people were frequently cast as dependent and burdensome, rather than as individuals with agency, expertise, and value.

This narrow focus also encouraged diagnostic overshadowing, where symptoms unrelated to a disability were wrongly attributed to it (Nami 2025; World Health Organization 2011). For instance, a person with an intellectual disability presenting with chest pain might be dismissed as "anxious" rather than being assessed for a heart condition. Such errors reflect the dangers of an overly medicalized perspective, where disability itself becomes a lens that distorts all clinical judgment.

The Social Model of Disability

The social model of disability, developed in the 1970s and 1980s by disabled activists and scholars, radically challenged the assumptions of the medical model (Oliver 1990; Charlton 1998). Instead of locating disability within the individual body, the social model argues that disability is created by society's failure to provide accessible environments and inclusive attitudes. In this view, people with impairments are only "disabled" because of barriers such as inaccessible transportation, discriminatory hiring practices, or stigmatizing stereotypes.

The social model reframed disability as a civil rights issue rather than a purely medical one (Charlton 1998; United Nations 2006). Its influence led to landmark policies such as the Americans with Disabilities Act (ADA) of 1990, which prohibited discrimination against people with disabilities in employment, public services, and healthcare. Globally, the United Nations' Convention on the Rights of Persons with Disabilities (CRPD) affirmed that disability justice is a matter of human rights and dignity, not charity or pity.

For nursing, the social model highlights the importance of addressing environmental and systemic barriers rather than focusing exclusively on "fixing" individuals (Oliver 1990; American Nurses Association 2015). A nurse who adopts this perspective may recognize that a patient's difficulty attending follow-up appointments stems not from "noncompliance" but from inaccessible public transportation. By shifting the locus of responsibility from the patient's body to society's structures, the social model opens new avenues for advocacy and patient-centered care.

The Biopsychosocial and Cultural Models

While the medical and social models are often presented in opposition, nursing practice frequently requires a more integrated approach (Engel 1977; Barnes and Mercer 2010). The biopsychosocial model, developed by George Engel in 1977, acknowledges that health and illness arise from the interplay of biological, psychological, and social factors. This model resonates strongly with nursing's holistic ethos, as it allows practitioners to attend simultaneously to physical impairments, mental health, and social context.

Additionally, the cultural model of disability emphasizes the ways in which cultural values and narratives shape understandings of disability (Barnes and Mercer 2010). For example, societies that prize independence and productivity may stigmatize those who require support, whereas collectivist cultures may view interdependence as a natural and valued aspect of community life. For nurses working in multicultural settings, awareness of cultural attitudes toward disability is essential to providing respectful and effective care.

Historical Marginalization of Disabled People

Theoretical models reflect but also shape societal attitudes (Barnes and Mercer 2010). Historically, disabled people have been subject to exclusion and mistreatment, often under the guise of care. In the late nineteenth and early twentieth centuries, institutionalization became a dominant response to disability. People with intellectual and developmental disabilities, psychiatric conditions, or physical impairments were frequently confined to asylums or custodial institutions, where neglect and abuse were common. Nurses working in these settings were often tasked with maintaining order rather than promoting autonomy or dignity.

The eugenics movement further reinforced ableist ideologies by promoting the sterilization and segregation of disabled individuals, with healthcare professionals—including nurses sometimes complicit in these practices (Barnes and Mercer 2010; Charlton 1998). This dark history underscores the importance of critically examining the role of healthcare in perpetuating injustice. Nurses must confront this legacy in order to avoid repeating it in subtler forms today.

The Disability Rights Movement and Nursing

The disability rights movement of the 1960s and 1970s paralleled other civil rights struggles, demanding equality, accessibility, and respect for disabled people (Charlton 1998; United Nations 2006). Activists insisted that "nothing about us without us," challenging the paternalism of medical professionals and calling for disabled people to have a voice in decisions affecting their lives. This movement led to major policy achievements, including the ADA, Section 504 of the Rehabilitation Act, and later, the CRPD.

Nursing has been both challenged and enriched by the disability rights movement (Charlton 1998; Nami 2025). Nurses, trained to advocate for patients, have had to reconcile their professional commitments with critiques from disabled activists who identified nursing and medicine as sources of oppression. This tension has pushed the profession toward greater humility and partnership, encouraging nurses to move from speaking for disabled patients to collaborating with them as partners in care.

Nursing Within Theoretical Frameworks

For nursing practice, the challenge lies in integrating these models and movements into everyday care (Engel 1977; American Nurses Association 2015). While the medical model remains necessary for addressing pain, illness, and rehabilitation, the social and cultural models remind nurses that disability is not solely a biological condition but also a social experience. The biopsychosocial model offers a practical framework for combining these perspectives, allowing nurses to provide holistic care while advocating for systemic change.

By embracing these frameworks, nurses can better identify and resist ableist assumptions in their practice (Nami 2025; Shakespeare 2013). They can move beyond viewing disability as a deficit to recognizing it as a form of human diversity. In doing so, they align their work with both the ethical mandates of the ANA and ICN and the aspirations of the disability rights movement.

Conceptual Analysis of Ableism in Nursing

A draft of my paper on ableism in healthcare serves as a foundation for this section, applying Walker and Avant's method of concept analysis to examine how the concept operates in nursing (Walker and Avant 2011; Nami 2025). Concept analysis is valuable because it provides a structured way to clarify abstract ideas, identify their defining features, and establish boundaries that distinguish them from related but distinct concepts. In the case of ableism, this process illuminates the ways in which disability-related discrimination functions within healthcare systems and nursing practice, often invisibly, yet with significant consequences for patients and providers alike.

Walker and Avant (2011) define "defining attributes" as the core characteristics that consistently appear when the concept is present. In the draft of my paper, several defining attributes of ableism in nursing are identified. One key attribute is the privileging of able-bodied norms, where "normal" health is equated with independence, productivity, and physical capacity, which, in turn, devalues those who cannot or do not conform to these standards (Nami 2025; Barnes and Mercer 2010). Another defining attribute is the stigmatization of difference, in which disabled bodies or minds are viewed as deviant, deficient, or undesirable. Ableism also manifests through exclusion and marginalization, where practices or policies deny disabled people full participation in healthcare and society. Additionally, the invisibility of disabled voices remains a critical concern, as decisions are often made about disabled individuals without their input, reinforcing paternalistic approaches to care.

These attributes demonstrate that ableism is not simply about negative attitudes toward disability, but also about the normalization of certain values, such as independence, productivity, and conformity, which marginalize those who do not embody them (Nami 2025; Shakespeare 2013). In nursing practice, this may appear in subtle ways, such as emphasizing recovery goals centered on independence in activities of daily living, even when patients may prioritize interdependence or community belonging.

Antecedents are events or circumstances that must occur before ableism can take shape (Walker and Avant 2011). In the draft of my paper, several antecedents are identified. Cultural ideals of productivity and independence position disabled individuals as less valuable within societal hierarchies (Barnes and Mercer 2010; Shakespeare 2013). The medicalization of disability, rooted in historical efforts to diagnose, treat, or "cure" impairments, frames disability as pathology (Oliver 1990; Shakespeare 2013). Historical legacies of institutionalization and eugenics have contributed to entrenched stigma that persists today (Barnes and Mercer 2010; Charlton 1998). Furthermore, ableism intersects with broader systems of oppression, including racism, sexism, and classism, resulting in compounded disadvantage (Charlton 1998; Garland-Thomson 2017). Within nursing, these antecedents shape curricula, clinical practice, and institutional priorities. For example, students may be trained to "fix" or "rehabilitate" rather than to understand and value diverse forms of embodiment and communication.

Consequences are the outcomes that result when the concept is present (Walker and Avant 2011). In healthcare and nursing, ableism produces both individual and systemic consequences. Disabled individuals experience poorer health outcomes, lower life expectancy, and higher rates of unmet healthcare needs (Buettner-Schmidt and Lobo 2012; World Health Organization 2011). Psychological harm is also significant, as repeated exposure to devaluation and exclusion contributes to increased stress, depression, and anxiety. Ableism may lead to delayed or inadequate care, particularly through diagnostic overshadowing and provider bias, resulting in missed diagnoses or inappropriate treatment. Over time, these experiences contribute to an erosion of trust, as patients who perceive discrimination may disengage from healthcare systems. Nurses themselves may also experience moral distress when they witness or participate in ableist practices, leading to ethical conflict and burnout. These consequences underscore that ableism is not an abstract concept but one with measurable and harmful effects on health and well-being (Buettner-Schmidt and Lobo 2012; World Health Organization 2011).

Empirical referents are measurable indicators that signal when the concept is present (Walker and Avant 2011). In the draft of my paper, examples include disparities in screening rates, such as lower rates of mammography, colonoscopy, and preventive care among disabled populations despite medical need (World Health Organization 2011). Accessibility audits also serve as indicators, revealing the absence of ramps, adaptive equipment, interpreters, or accessible exam tables in clinical environments. Patient-reported experiences provide additional evidence, with surveys and qualitative studies documenting dismissal, disrespect, or exclusion. Workforce demographics further highlight systemic inequities, as individuals with disabilities remain underrepresented among healthcare professionals. These referents provide concrete ways to measure ableism and to identify gaps in care, allowing for the evaluation of progress over time (Walker and Avant 2011; Nami 2025).

Walker and Avant (2011) also emphasize the importance of model, borderline, and contrary cases in clarifying conceptual boundaries. A model case of ableism in nursing involves a nurse who assumes that a patient with cerebral palsy presenting with abdominal pain is experiencing chronic discomfort related to their disability, and therefore fails to order appropriate diagnostic tests. The patient is later diagnosed with appendicitis that could have been treated earlier, illustrating stigmatization, diagnostic overshadowing, and exclusion from appropriate care (Nami 2025). A borderline case involves a patient with a mobility impairment who is scheduled for physical therapy to regain independence. While the plan reflects the privileging of independence as a norm, the therapy aligns with the patient's goals and consent, demonstrating only partial features of ableism. A contrary case illustrates anti-ableist practice, where a deaf patient is admitted to a hospital and the nursing team immediately arranges for a certified ASL interpreter, provides accessible written materials, and ensures full inclusion in decision-making processes. These cases illustrate how ableism can manifest across a spectrum, from overt discrimination to subtle bias and, ultimately, to inclusive and equitable care (Walker and Avant 2011; Nami 2025).

The draft of my paper underscores that ableism, as clarified through concept analysis, is not an abstract concept but one with direct implications for nursing education, practice, and policy (Nami 2025; Walker and Avant 2011). By identifying defining attributes, antecedents, consequences, and empirical referents, nurses can more readily recognize ableism when it occurs. Model cases highlight the urgency of intervention, while contrary cases demonstrate what anti-ableist care can look like in practice.

Ultimately, the value of this analysis lies in its capacity to move nursing beyond unexamined assumptions (Nami 2025). By naming and clarifying ableism, the profession can more effectively design interventions that dismantle its presence in healthcare systems, from clinical care to institutional policy.

Ableism in Nursing Education and Practice

While the draft of my paper provides a conceptual foundation for understanding ableism, the next step is to examine how this discrimination manifests concretely in nursing education and practice (Nami 2025). Nurses are at the frontlines of healthcare delivery, and their attitudes, training, and institutional environments profoundly shape the quality of care patients receive. Unfortunately, ableism continues to influence nursing curricula, professional norms, and day-to-day care, perpetuating disparities and undermining the values of equity and holistic practice.

Ableism in Nursing Education

Nursing education is critical to shaping the worldview of future practitioners (American Nurses Association 2015). However, curricula often reinforce ableist assumptions, either by omission or through an overemphasis on the medical model of disability. Students are frequently taught to approach disability primarily as a set of pathologies to be managed or corrected, rather than as a lived experience shaped by social and environmental factors.

For example, textbooks may describe conditions in terms of deficits and burdens, using language that frames disability as tragic or undesirable (Barnes and Mercer 2010; Garland-Thomson 2017). Case studies often position nondisabled functioning as the goal of care, ignoring alternative frameworks of interdependence or accommodation. In clinical placements, students may see disabled patients treated as passive recipients of care, with limited opportunities to participate in decision-making. These educational patterns reinforce paternalistic attitudes and discourage the recognition of disabled individuals as partners in their own care.

Another major gap lies in the limited inclusion of disability studies perspectives in nursing curricula (Nami 2025). While diversity and cultural competency training often address race, ethnicity, and gender, disability is less frequently integrated. This absence leaves students ill prepared to identify or challenge ableism in practice. As a result, new nurses may unconsciously perpetuate biases or fail to recognize the structural barriers disabled patients face.

Disabled students in nursing programs face their own unique challenges (Nami 2025). Many encounter physical barriers in labs or classrooms, lack of accommodations during clinical placements, or stigma from faculty and peers who doubt their capacity to practice. These barriers reflect the profession's historic reluctance to embrace disability within its own ranks, a reluctance that perpetuates ableism by limiting the diversity of voices in nursing itself.

Implicit Bias and Attitudes Toward Disability

Beyond formal education, implicit bias plays a powerful role in shaping how nurses perceive and interact with disabled patients (Nami 2025; World Health Organization 2011). Research has shown that healthcare providers often harbor unconscious assumptions that disabled individuals have a lower quality of life, are less capable of making decisions, or require less aggressive care. Such attitudes can subtly influence everything from the tone of communication to the willingness to pursue complex treatments.

One striking example is diagnostic overshadowing, a phenomenon in which new or unrelated health concerns are wrongly attributed to a person's existing disability (Nami 2025). For instance, a patient with an intellectual disability who reports pain may be dismissed as "acting out" rather than evaluated for an underlying condition. Similarly, a person with a mobility impairment might have fatigue or shortness of breath attributed to "deconditioning" when it is actually cardiac disease. These patterns are not only dismissive but dangerous, as they delay timely diagnosis and treatment.

Bias also affects communication (Nami 2025). Patients who use augmentative communication devices, interpreters, or alternative methods of expression may encounter impatience or frustration from providers, leading to rushed interactions and inadequate explanations. In these cases, ableism undermines the ethical principle of informed consent by denying patients the opportunity to fully understand and participate in their care.

Systemic Barriers in Clinical Practice

Ableism in nursing is not only a matter of individual bias but also of systemic structures that disadvantage disabled patients (World Health Organization 2011; Nami 2025). Many healthcare facilities remain physically inaccessible, with exam tables, diagnostic equipment, and restrooms not designed for individuals with mobility limitations. Policies may not account for the additional time or resources required to provide equitable care, leaving nurses constrained by productivity standards that privilege efficiency over accessibility.

Time pressures, staffing shortages, and electronic documentation requirements also contribute to systemic ableism (Nami 2025). Nurses working under strict schedules may feel unable to allocate the extra time required to support patients with communication needs, mobility challenges, or complex conditions. When institutions fail to account for these realities, patients bear the burden of exclusion.

Structural ableism also intersects with insurance and healthcare financing (World Health Organization 2011). Disabled patients may be denied coverage for necessary supports, such as home healthcare or durable medical equipment, because such services are considered "nonessential." Nurses often witness the harm caused by these denials but may feel powerless to intervene. This tension contributes to moral distress among providers and perpetuates inequities in care.

Paternalism and the Denial of Autonomy

One of the most persistent forms of ableism in practice is paternalism, in which nurses and other providers assume that they know what is best for disabled patients, regardless of the patients' own expressed wishes (Charlton 1998; American Nurses Association 2015). This can manifest in subtle ways, such as speaking to a caregiver instead of the patient, or in overt ways, such as disregarding a patient's refusal of treatment.

Paternalism undermines autonomy and dignity, two principles central to nursing ethics (American Nurses Association 2015). It also ignores the reality that disabled people are often experts in their own bodies and conditions, with years of lived experience managing symptoms, navigating systems, and identifying effective strategies. By disregarding this expertise, nursing practice risks alienating patients and perpetuating inequities.

Implications for Nursing Practice

The presence of ableism in nursing education and practice has profound implications (Nami 2025). It shapes how nurses are trained, how they perceive patients, and how healthcare institutions deliver services. Left unaddressed, it perpetuates health disparities, undermines trust, and conflicts with the profession's ethical commitments.

Addressing these issues requires more than individual awareness (Nami 2025). It demands structural reforms in curricula, institutional policies, and professional culture. Nursing education must incorporate disability justice perspectives, ensuring students understand both the historical oppression of disabled people and the principles of anti-ableist care. Clinical settings must be restructured to promote accessibility, provide adequate resources, and support nurses in offering inclusive care. Above all, the profession must recognize ableism as a form of systemic oppression that is as urgent and harmful as racism, sexism, or classism.

Introduction to the Neurodiversity Paradigm

The neurodiversity paradigm represents a significant shift in how differences in cognition, behavior, and neurological functioning are understood within both society and healthcare (Singer 1999; Blume 1998). Emerging from the disability rights movement and popularized in the late 1990s by sociologist Judy Singer, the concept of neurodiversity reframes conditions such as autism, ADHD, dyslexia, and other neurodevelopmental differences not as deficits or pathologies, but as natural variations of the human mind. This paradigm challenges long-standing biomedical assumptions that equate difference with disorder and instead emphasizes diversity, inclusion, and respect for neurological variation.

Within traditional healthcare frameworks, neurodevelopmental conditions have largely been interpreted through a deficit-based lens (Nami 2025). Diagnostic criteria, treatment goals, and care plans have historically centered on normalization reducing symptoms, increasing conformity to social norms, and promoting independence as defined by dominant cultural expectations. While these approaches have led to important supports and interventions, they have also contributed to the marginalization of neurodivergent individuals by framing their ways of thinking and being as inherently inferior.

The neurodiversity paradigm offers an alternative perspective (Singer 1999; Blume 1998). It asserts that neurological differences are part of the natural spectrum of human diversity, similar to variations in race, culture, or language. Rather than asking how individuals can be made more "normal," this paradigm asks how environments, systems, and social expectations can be adapted to be more inclusive. For nursing, which emphasizes holistic, patient-centered care, this shift has profound implications. It requires moving beyond deficit-based models and toward an approach that recognizes neurodivergent individuals as whole persons with strengths, preferences, and agency.

Importantly, neurodiversity does not deny the challenges associated with certain conditions (Singer 1999). Many neurodivergent individuals experience significant difficulties related to sensory processing, communication, executive functioning, or co-occurring medical and psychiatric conditions. However, the paradigm distinguishes between impairment and oppression, recognizing that many of the difficulties faced by neurodivergent individuals arise not solely from their neurological differences, but from environments that are inaccessible, rigid, or unaccommodating. This distinction aligns closely with the social model of disability and reinforces the argument that ableism, rather than difference itself, is a primary driver of inequity.

Historical and Theoretical Foundations of Neurodiversity Paradigm

The neurodiversity paradigm emerged at the intersection of disability activism, sociology, and lived experience (Singer 1999; Blume 1998). Judy Singer introduced the term "neurodiversity" to challenge the dominant narratives surrounding autism and to advocate for recognition of neurological differences as a form of diversity rather than deficit. Around the same time, journalist Harvey Blume helped popularize the concept, emphasizing its relevance to broader cultural and technological shifts.

The paradigm is deeply rooted in the social model of disability, which reframes disability as a product of societal barriers rather than individual impairment (Oliver

1990). However, neurodiversity extends this model by emphasizing identity, culture, and community. For many individuals, particularly within the autistic community, neurodivergence is not simply a condition to be managed but an integral part of identity. This perspective has given rise to concepts such as neurodivergent culture, self-advocacy, and the rejection of language that frames individuals as "broken" or "defective."

The neurodiversity paradigm also intersects with critical disability studies, which examine how power, language, and institutions shape understandings of normality and difference (Garland-Thomson 2017; Barnes and Mercer 2010). From this perspective, diagnostic categories are not neutral descriptors but are embedded within systems that prioritize certain ways of thinking and functioning over others. For example, traits such as direct communication, intense focus, or sensory sensitivity often associated with autism may be pathologized in clinical contexts but valued in other environments. This highlights the contextual nature of disability and underscores the importance of examining how societal norms define and enforce "normality."

Within nursing, these theoretical developments challenge traditional frameworks that prioritize independence, productivity, and normative functioning (Nami 2025; Singer 1999). They call into question whether commonly accepted goals such as promoting independence in activities of daily living are universally appropriate or whether they reflect culturally specific values that may not align with patients' lived experiences or preferences. By engaging with the neurodiversity paradigm, nursing can begin to critically examine its own assumptions and expand its understanding of what constitutes health, well-being, and quality of life.

Disability Rights and Advocacy in Nursing

The fight against ableism in healthcare cannot be separated from the broader struggle for disability rights (Americans with Disabilities Act 1990; United Nations 2006). Legal, cultural, and political movements have pushed societies to recognize disabled people as full citizens entitled to dignity, autonomy, and equality. These changes have reshaped the context in which nurses practice, providing frameworks that both challenge and guide the profession. For nursing, understanding disability rights is not just a matter of compliance with laws but an ethical imperative grounded in advocacy, justice, and the promotion of health equity.

The Americans with Disabilities Act (ADA)

The ADA of 1990 was a landmark in disability rights legislation in the United States, prohibiting discrimination in employment, public services, and healthcare (Americans with Disabilities Act 1990). For nursing, the ADA carries several direct implications: healthcare facilities must ensure physical accessibility, provide reasonable accommodations, and communicate effectively with patients who have disabilities. This includes ensuring that exam tables are height-adjustable, interpreters are available for patients who are deaf or hard of hearing, and written materials are provided in accessible formats.

Despite these requirements, compliance is uneven (World Health Organization 2011; Nami 2025). Many facilities remain inaccessible, interpreters are not consistently provided, and communication accommodations are treated as optional rather than essential. Nurses are often the first to witness the consequences of these gaps, as patients encounter preventable barriers that compromise their care. In such cases, nurses act not only as caregivers but as advocates who must press institutions to honor their obligations under the law.

The Convention on the Rights of Persons with Disabilities (CRPD)

Globally, the United Nations Convention on the Rights of Persons with Disabilities (CRPD), adopted in 2006, has reinforced the principle that disability rights are human rights (United Nations 2006). Unlike the ADA, which is primarily anti-discrimination law, the CRPD provides a holistic vision of inclusion, requiring states to promote participation, accessibility, and autonomy across all aspects of life.

For nursing, the CRPD emphasizes a shift away from charity or medicalized models of disability toward recognition of agency, equality, and self-determination (United Nations 2006; Charlton 1998). This means nurses must not only provide care but also support the full social inclusion of disabled individuals. For example, respecting a patient's right to make informed decisions about their care even when those decisions challenge medical advice aligns with the CRPD's emphasis on autonomy and dignity.

Although the United States has signed but not ratified the CRPD, its principles have influenced global nursing education and advocacy (United Nations 2006). International nursing organizations increasingly frame disability as an equity issue, recognizing that ableism undermines health on a global scale.

Disability Pride and Cultural Humility

Legal frameworks like the ADA and CRPD establish rights, but cultural shifts are equally important for dismantling ableism in healthcare (Americans with Disabilities Act 1990; United Nations 2006). Movements such as Disability Pride emphasize that disability is not merely an individual impairment but a valued aspect of human diversity. Disability Pride challenges the notion that disabled lives are tragic, instead affirming resilience, creativity, and community.

For nursing, adopting a Disability Pride perspective means valuing patients not despite their disabilities but in recognition of the strengths and perspectives disability brings (Garland-Thomson 2017; Charlton 1998). It requires moving away from "fixing" patients toward supporting them in achieving their own goals of health, autonomy, and inclusion.

Closely related is the concept of cultural humility. Unlike cultural competency, which suggests mastery of knowledge about different groups, cultural humility emphasizes lifelong learning, reflection, and partnership (Nami 2025). Nurses practicing cultural humility with disabled patients acknowledge the limits of their expertise, honor the authority of lived experience, and remain open to correction and growth. This approach shifts power dynamics, placing patients at the center of care.

Nursing as Policy Advocates

Nurses are uniquely positioned to advocate for disability rights, both at the bedside and at the policy level (American Nurses Association 2015; United Nations 2006). Their proximity to patients gives them firsthand insight into the barriers disabled people face, from inaccessible facilities to gaps in insurance coverage. Yet advocacy requires moving beyond individual problem-solving toward systemic change.

Professional nursing organizations, such as the American Nurses Association (ANA), have called for equitable healthcare policies and inclusive practices (American Nurses Association 2015). Nurses can contribute by joining policy committees, lobbying for legislation that expands access to care, and ensuring that disability rights are central to health equity initiatives. On a smaller scale, nurses can advocate within their institutions for accessibility audits, disability-inclusive curricula, and recruitment of disabled professionals into the nursing workforce.

Nursing practice requires that without systemic advocacy, ableism will continue to undermine patient outcomes (Nami 2025). For example, without policy reform, insurance systems may continue to deny coverage for essential supports like personal care attendants, durable medical equipment, or mental health services. Nurses can amplify patient voices in these debates, ensuring that policy decisions reflect the lived realities of disabled people.

Intersectionality in Advocacy

Disability rights advocacy in nursing must also account for intersectionality (Charlton 1998; Garland-Thomson 2017). Disabled people of color, LGBTQ+ individuals with disabilities, and low-income disabled populations experience unique barriers that cannot be addressed by disability policy alone. Addressing disparities requires cross-movement solidarity, linking disability justice with racial justice, gender equity, and LGBTQ+ rights.

Nurses can serve as bridge-builders in this work, fostering coalitions that recognize the complexity of patients' lives (American Nurses Association 2015; Charlton 1998). Advocacy rooted in intersectionality aligns with the profession's holistic approach, ensuring that care and policy address the whole person rather than isolated aspects of identity.

From Advocacy to Action

Ultimately, disability rights advocacy in nursing requires a shift from passive acknowledgment to active engagement (American Nurses Association 2015; Charlton 1998). Nurses must see themselves not only as caregivers but as agents of change within healthcare systems. This includes the following:

- Demanding accessibility in clinical settings (Americans with Disabilities Act 1990).
- Challenging paternalistic practices that undermine autonomy.
- Incorporating disability perspectives into curricula and research.
- Supporting legislation that expands equity and inclusion.

Such actions affirm nursing's ethical commitments while also addressing the systemic roots of ableism (American Nurses Association 2015; Nami 2025). By aligning their practice with disability rights frameworks, nurses move closer to fulfilling the profession's mission of promoting health, dignity, and justice for all.

Strategies for Anti-Ableist Nursing

Recognizing ableism in nursing is only the beginning; the greater challenge lies in dismantling it and reimagining how care is taught, delivered, and evaluated (Nami 2025). Anti-ableist nursing requires a sustained commitment to reshaping education, transforming clinical practice, producing evidence through research, advocating for policy reform, and fostering a culture of reflection and accountability.

One of the most pressing areas for reform is nursing education (Nami 2025). The ways in which students are trained directly influence how they will interact with disabled patients in the future. Traditionally, nursing curricula have focused on the medical aspects of disability, emphasizing diagnosis, pathology, and rehabilitation. While these are important areas of knowledge, they risk reducing disabled individuals to conditions rather than whole persons with unique experiences and strengths. Integrating disability justice frameworks into curricula can help counter this imbalance, presenting disability not only as a clinical phenomenon but also as a social, cultural, and political reality.

Students should encounter disabled educators, activists, and patients in their training, whose lived experiences provide critical perspectives often absent from textbooks (Charlton 1998; Nami 2025). Case studies can be redesigned to highlight the dangers of ableist assumptions and to illustrate the value of inclusive care planning. Furthermore, training must emphasize intersectionality, teaching students to understand how disability interacts with race, gender, and class to shape health outcomes. Nursing education must also become more inclusive for students with disabilities themselves, ensuring that they receive accommodations, mentorship, and equal opportunities to succeed. Their presence in the profession is itself a powerful counter to ableist assumptions about who can and cannot be a nurse.

In practice, anti-ableist nursing requires reimagining the everyday delivery of care (Nami 2025). One important approach is the adoption of universal design principles in healthcare environments. When spaces and systems are designed to be accessible from the outset through features, such as adjustable exam tables, wide doorways, accessible signage, and simplified documentation processes, they benefit not only disabled patients but the entire patient population. Accessible communication is another vital dimension of inclusive practice. Nurses must be prepared to use interpreters, plain language, and assistive technology to ensure that patients fully understand their care and can participate in decision-making. Equitable care also depends on rethinking how time is valued. Institutional pressures to maximize efficiency often disadvantage patients with communication or mobility challenges, who may require more time to be fully supported. Anti-ableist practice insists that such time is not an inefficiency but an essential part of equitable care. At the heart of this approach is shared decision-making, which recognizes that disabled patients are experts in their own lives. By valuing their preferences and lived expertise, nurses move away from paternalism and toward true partnership.

Research provides another crucial tool for dismantling ableism (Nami 2025). Nursing scholarship must document how disabled people experience care, measure the impact of ableist structures, and test interventions designed to counter discrimination. For example, studies can evaluate the effects of redesigned curricula, accessibility audits, or community-based participatory research projects in which disabled individuals act not as subjects but as co-researchers. Empirical evidence of disparities in preventive screenings, pain management, or health outcomes can be used to push institutions toward accountability. Research should also address intersectionality, recognizing that the effects of ableism are magnified when combined with racism, sexism, or poverty. By producing robust evidence, nursing research strengthens advocacy and guides the development of effective anti-ableist strategies.

Policy advocacy is equally important (American Nurses Association 2015). Nurses have long been trusted voices in debates over health and equity, and they can use this influence to press for reforms that address systemic ableism. Policy changes might include expanding insurance coverage for home health services and durable medical equipment, strengthening enforcement of accessibility laws, or embedding disability equity into accreditation standards for healthcare organizations. At the workforce level, advocacy is needed to recruit and retain nurses with disabilities, ensuring that the profession itself becomes more representative of the communities it serves. Nursing organizations can amplify these efforts by placing disability rights at the center of their equity agendas, lobbying for legislation that supports inclusion, and ensuring that disabled people are represented in decision-making.

Finally, anti-ableist nursing requires a cultural shift toward reflection and accountability (Nami 2025). Nurses and institutions must embrace cultural humility, a practice that emphasizes lifelong learning and openness to correction. Creating forums where nurses can reflect on their biases, share ethical dilemmas, and learn from disabled colleagues and patients is essential. Institutions should establish accountability mechanisms such as patient advisory councils, accessibility reviews, and transparent reporting processes for discrimination. Beyond compliance, nursing must actively celebrate disability as a valued aspect of human diversity, highlighting the strengths, creativity, and expertise that disabled patients and professionals bring to healthcare.

Taken together, these strategies make clear that anti-ableist nursing is not a matter of individual goodwill but a systemic transformation (Nami 2025). Education must be restructured, clinical practices redesigned, research expanded, policies reformed, and professional cultures shifted. Such changes require persistence and courage, as they call into question long-standing assumptions and practices. Yet they are essential for fulfilling nursing's mission: to advocate for dignity, promote equity, and provide holistic care for all people.

Conclusion

Ableism remains one of the most overlooked yet pervasive barriers in healthcare (Nami 2025; World Health Organization 2011). For too long, nursing has operated within systems and assumptions that treat disability as a deviation from "normal" rather than as a natural and valuable form of human diversity. This chapter has examined ableism from multiple perspectives—conceptual, historical, educational, clinical, and policy-based—demonstrating how deeply embedded it is in nursing practice and how urgent it is to address.

The draft of my paper provided a conceptual framework for analyzing ableism, identifying its defining attributes, antecedents, consequences, and empirical referents (Walker and Avant 2011; Nami 2025). This analysis revealed that ableism is not limited to overt discrimination but is often woven into the very fabric of healthcare delivery, shaping how patients are perceived, how care is prioritized, and how systems are structured. It also highlighted the importance of distinguishing between model cases, which fully reflect the harm of ableist assumptions, and contrary cases, which demonstrate what anti-ableist care can look like in practice.

Historically, nursing has been shaped by the medical model of disability, which has contributed to important advances but has also reinforced the idea that disabled bodies are inherently deficient (Oliver 1990; Shakespeare 2013). The social model of disability, alongside disability rights movements and legislative milestones such as the ADA and CRPD, has challenged this perspective, emphasizing that disability arises as much from social and environmental barriers as from individual impairments. For nursing, adopting these alternative frameworks shifts the focus from "fixing" patients to dismantling barriers and supporting autonomy, dignity, and inclusion.

The analysis of nursing education and practice underscored the persistence of ableism in curricula, clinical training, and professional culture (Nami 2025). From diagnostic overshadowing to paternalism, ableism continues to undermine patient autonomy and contribute to health disparities. Yet these challenges also highlight opportunities for reform. Nursing education can incorporate disability justice perspectives, support disabled students, and prepare future nurses to recognize and challenge bias. Clinical practice can be redesigned to reflect universal design principles, prioritize accessible communication, and treat time as an equity tool rather than a productivity cost. Research can measure ableism and test interventions, while policy advocacy can secure systemic reforms that extend beyond individual encounters.

In addition, the integration of the neurodiversity paradigm in nursing education further deepens this call to action by challenging nursing to reconsider not only how disability is treated, but how difference itself is understood (Singer 1999; Blume 1998). Neurodiversity exposes the limitations of deficit-based frameworks that continue to shape clinical practice, education, and policy, revealing how deeply assumptions about normality, independence, and productivity are embedded within the profession. By recognizing neurodivergent individuals as experts in their own experiences and as contributors to human diversity rather than deviations from it, nursing is compelled to move beyond accommodation toward genuine inclusion. This shift is not merely conceptual but transformative: it demands that healthcare systems, environments, and professional norms be redesigned to support a wider range of cognitive and behavioral expressions. In embracing neurodiversity, nursing does not abandon its commitment to alleviating suffering, but rather strengthens it by ensuring that care is guided not by conformity, but by respect, partnership, and equity.

At every stage, anti-ableist nursing requires humility, reflection, and accountability (Nami 2025). Nurses must recognize the limitations of their own perspectives and remain open to learning from disabled patients, colleagues, and communities. Cultural humility ensures that anti-ableist practice is not a one-time adjustment but a lifelong commitment to inclusion and justice. The profession must also move beyond individual awareness to collective action, demanding structural reforms that eliminate systemic barriers and build equity into the very design of healthcare systems.

The conclusion is clear: dismantling ableism is not peripheral to nursing but central to its mission (American Nurses Association 2015; Nami 2025). Nursing's commitment to human dignity, equity, and holistic care cannot be realized without addressing the discrimination and exclusion that disabled people continue to face. Nurses must embrace their role not only as caregivers but as advocates and change agents, working to transform education, practice, policy, and culture.

The future of nursing depends on this commitment (Nami 2025). A truly inclusive and just healthcare system will emerge only when nurses actively resist ableism, amplify the voices of disabled people, and reimagine care as a partnership grounded in respect and equity. By doing so, the profession can move closer to fulfilling its highest ethical obligations and contribute to a healthcare system that honors the dignity and diversity of all human lives.

References

American Nurses Association. Code of ethics for nurses with interpretive statements. ANA; 2015.
Americans with Disabilities Act of 1990, Pub. L. No. 101-336, 104 Stat. 328. 1990.
Barnes C, Mercer G. Exploring disability. 2nd ed. Polity Press; 2010.

Blume H. Neurodiversity. The Atlantic. 1998. https://www.theatlantic.com/magazine/archive/1998/09/neurodiversity/305909/.

Buettner-Schmidt K, Lobo ML. Social justice: a concept analysis. J Adv Nurs. 2012;68(4):948–58. https://doi.org/10.1111/j.1365-2648.2011.05856.x.

Charlton JI. Nothing about us without us: disability oppression and empowerment. University of California Press; 1998.

Engel GL. The need for a new medical model: a challenge for biomedicine. Science. 1977;196(4286):129–36. https://doi.org/10.1126/science.847460.

Garland-Thomson R. Disability bioethics: toward a new discourse of human value. Hastings Cent Rep. 2017;47(3):4–9. https://doi.org/10.1002/hast.718.

Nami N. Ableism: a concept analysis in nursing. Unpublished manuscript. University of Missouri–Kansas City; 2025.

Oliver M. The politics of disablement. Macmillan; 1990.

Shakespeare T. Disability rights and wrongs revisited. 2nd ed. Routledge; 2013.

Singer J. Why can't you be normal for once in your life? From a "problem with no name" to the emergence of a new category of difference. Honours thesis. University of Technology Sydney; 1999.

United Nations. Convention on the rights of persons with disabilities. 2006. https://www.un.org/disabilities/documents/convention/convoptprot-e.pdf.

Walker LO, Avant KC. Strategies for theory construction in nursing. 5th ed. Prentice Hall; 2011.

World Health Organization. World report on disability. WHO Press; 2011.

Racial Disparities in Nursing 3

Introduction to Racial Disparities

The nursing profession is guided by values of compassion, respect, and justice, yet it does not operate in a vacuum (American Nurses Association 2015). Like all areas of healthcare, nursing exists within a society that is profoundly shaped by systemic racism. The persistence of racial disparities in both health outcomes and access to care underscores how inequities are woven into the very fabric of the US healthcare system. For nurses, who occupy one of the most trusted roles in society, addressing these disparities is not optional but essential to upholding the profession's ethical obligations.

Racial disparities in healthcare can be defined as systematic differences in health outcomes, healthcare access, and treatment experiences among racial and ethnic groups (Institute of Medicine 2003; Bailey et al. 2017). These disparities are not attributable to biological differences between groups but are instead rooted in historical, social, economic, and political inequities. The Centers for Disease Control and Prevention (CDC) defines health disparities as "preventable differences in the burden of disease, injury, violence, or opportunities to achieve optimal health that are experienced by socially disadvantaged populations." Within this framework, race functions as a social construct that has been used to distribute privilege to some groups while producing disadvantage and harm for others.

It is important to distinguish between inequality and inequity (Bailey et al. 2017; Yearby 2020). Inequality refers simply to differences in outcomes, while inequity implies that those differences are unfair, unjust, and avoidable. For example, the fact that Black women in the United States are three to four times more likely to die during childbirth than White women is not an unfortunate coincidence, but a reflection of systemic inequities embedded in healthcare delivery, access, and bias. Recognizing inequity requires naming racism as a driver of poor outcomes, rather than attributing disparities to individual behaviors or choices.

N. Nami, *Unraveling Social Justice Issues in Nursing*,
https://doi.org/10.1007/978-3-032-26512-8_3

Historical context is essential for understanding racial disparities in nursing and healthcare more broadly (Smedley et al. 2003; Bailey et al. 2017). The legacy of slavery, segregation, and exclusion continues to shape health systems today. Hospitals in the United States were racially segregated well into the twentieth century, with Black patients often relegated to underfunded facilities or denied care altogether. The infamous Tuskegee Syphilis Study, in which treatment was deliberately withheld from Black men to study the natural progression of the disease, remains a stark reminder of how medical research has exploited and dehumanized communities of color. Such histories contribute not only to current inequities but also to mistrust of the healthcare system among marginalized populations.

Nursing itself has not been immune to racism (Bailey et al. 2017; American Nurses Association 2015). Historically, nursing schools excluded Black, Indigenous, and other minority students, limiting their entry into the profession. Even after integration, nurses of color often faced discrimination, from being tracked into less prestigious specialties to being denied promotions or leadership roles. The underrepresentation of racial and ethnic minorities in the nursing workforce continues to limit diversity in perspectives and leadership, perpetuating disparities in both education and patient care.

In patient care, racial disparities are evident across nearly every domain of health (CDC 2017; Institute of Medicine 2003). Black Americans face higher rates of hypertension, diabetes, stroke, and premature death compared to their White counterparts. Indigenous populations experience disproportionately high rates of suicide, substance use disorders, and chronic diseases, while Hispanic and Latino communities encounter barriers to preventive care and higher rates of certain occupational health risks. Asian American and Pacific Islander populations, though often portrayed through the "model minority" stereotype, also experience disparities, particularly in mental health access and culturally competent care. These patterns reflect the cumulative impact of systemic racism, social determinants of health, and healthcare discrimination.

The COVID-19 pandemic brought renewed attention to these disparities, as communities of color experienced disproportionately high rates of infection, hospitalization, and death (CDC 2021; Bailey et al. 2017). Structural inequities such as crowded housing, frontline employment, limited access to healthcare, and preexisting health disparities converged to create devastating outcomes. For nurses working on the frontlines of the pandemic, these inequities were impossible to ignore. The pandemic reinforced the reality that racial disparities are not isolated or occasional, but enduring and systemic.

Addressing racial disparities in nursing requires an honest appraisal of the ways racism shapes both the profession and the broader healthcare system (Bailey et al. 2017; Yearby 2020). It involves moving beyond cultural competency to cultural humility, which acknowledges the limits of one's knowledge and emphasizes continuous learning, reflection, and partnership with patients. It also demands an intersectional approach that recognizes how race interacts with class, gender, disability, and immigration status to compound disadvantage.

This chapter will examine racial disparities in nursing in depth, beginning with disparities in the nursing workforce and extending to disparities in patient care; will explore how systemic racism is reproduced through institutional policies, clinical algorithms, and workplace cultures; and will also highlight strategies for building an anti-racist nursing profession (Bailey et al. 2017; Yearby 2020). By situating these disparities within both historical and contemporary contexts, the chapter underscores that racial inequities in health are not inevitable but are the result of structures that can and must be dismantled.

Racial Disparities in the Nursing Workforce

While much attention is given to racial disparities in patient outcomes, inequities are also deeply rooted within the nursing workforce itself (Bailey et al. 2017; National Academies of Sciences, Engineering, and Medicine 2019). The nursing profession, often celebrated for its inclusivity and commitment to service, has historically excluded and marginalized nurses of color. These patterns remain visible today in the underrepresentation of minority groups in nursing, persistent workplace discrimination, and limited opportunities for advancement into leadership positions. Understanding these disparities is critical because the diversity of the nursing workforce directly impacts the quality, equity, and cultural responsiveness of patient care.

The demographics of nursing reveal clear disparities in representation (National Academies of Sciences, Engineering, and Medicine 2019). Although the United States is becoming increasingly diverse, the nursing workforce does not reflect this shift. According to the National Council of State Boards of Nursing, the majority of registered nurses identify as White, with Black, Hispanic/Latino, Indigenous, and Asian nurses making up a much smaller proportion of the workforce compared to their representation in the general population. This lack of diversity limits the profession's ability to meet the cultural and linguistic needs of patients, especially in underserved communities. It also reduces the availability of role models for aspiring nurses of color, perpetuating a cycle of underrepresentation.

The barriers begin early, in access to nursing education (Smedley et al. 2003; National Academies of Sciences, Engineering, and Medicine 2019). Historically, many nursing schools excluded Black and Indigenous students altogether, forcing the establishment of separate institutions such as historically Black nursing programs. Although overt exclusion is no longer permitted, subtle barriers continue to affect admissions and retention. Students of color often face financial hardship, lack of mentorship, and experiences of bias or stereotyping in academic settings. Language barriers can affect immigrant students, while structural inequities in primary and secondary education leave some applicants less prepared for the rigorous academic requirements of nursing school. Faculty diversity is also limited, which means students of color frequently lack mentors who share their cultural or racial background.

Even when nurses of color enter the workforce, they encounter discrimination in hiring, promotion, and daily interactions (Bailey et al. 2017; Williams and Mohammed 2013). Studies consistently show that nurses of color are less likely to be promoted into leadership or managerial roles compared to their White counterparts, even when qualifications are comparable. Pay disparities also persist, with Black and Hispanic nurses often earning less than White nurses for the same work. Discrimination is not only structural but also interpersonal, manifesting in microaggressions, exclusion from professional networks, and biased assumptions about competence. For example, nurses of color report being mistaken for non-professional staff, facing scrutiny over their language skills, or being excluded from collaborative decision-making processes.

Racism in the workplace is not limited to colleagues; it also arises in interactions with patients and families (Cuevas et al. 2019; Bailey et al. 2017). Nurses of color often experience patients refusing care from them on the basis of race or making overtly racist remarks. These encounters take a toll on nurses' psychological well-being and contribute to burnout, stress, and decreased job satisfaction. Without strong institutional support, nurses of color may feel isolated or undervalued, which affects not only their careers but also the quality of care delivered to patients. When racism is tolerated or inadequately addressed within healthcare organizations, it creates environments that are not only harmful to staff but also to the patients who depend on them.

Representation in leadership remains a critical gap (National Academies of Sciences, Engineering, and Medicine 2019). Nursing leadership, whether at the institutional, state, or national level, is overwhelmingly White. This lack of diversity has real consequences for policy, practice, and advocacy, as decision-making bodies often fail to reflect the perspectives and needs of minority nurses and the communities they serve. Efforts to address disparities in patient care will remain incomplete if the voices of nurses of color are not present in leadership roles. Moreover, diverse leadership fosters more inclusive workplaces, supports mentorship opportunities, and helps to dismantle structural barriers.

The consequences of workforce disparities extend beyond the profession itself (Institute of Medicine 2003; National Academies of Sciences, Engineering, and Medicine 2019). Patients often benefit from receiving care from providers who share their cultural or linguistic background, as this enhances trust, communication, and satisfaction with care. When the nursing workforce does not reflect the populations it serves, these opportunities for culturally concordant care are diminished. Research has shown that patients are more likely to adhere to treatment plans, report positive care experiences, and feel respected when they receive care from providers who understand their cultural context. Thus, racial disparities in the nursing workforce have direct implications for patient outcomes.

To address these inequities, nursing must confront both structural and cultural barriers within the profession (American Nurses Association 2015; Bailey et al. 2017). Recruitment efforts must be coupled with retention strategies, ensuring that nurses of color not only enter the field but thrive within it. This requires mentorship programs, financial support, inclusive curricula, and institutional policies that actively challenge discrimination. Nursing education must prioritize diversity in admissions, provide culturally responsive support services, and promote faculty diversity. In the workplace, organizations must adopt zero-tolerance policies for racism, provide ongoing training on bias and equity, and ensure transparency in promotion and pay practices.

Ultimately, racial disparities in the nursing workforce reflect larger societal inequities (Bailey et al. 2017; Yearby 2020). However, the nursing profession has the power and responsibility to lead by example. By creating a more diverse and equitable workforce, nursing can enhance patient care, strengthen the profession, and model the values of justice and inclusion it professes to uphold. Achieving this goal requires commitment at every level from academic institutions and healthcare organizations to professional associations and policy makers. Nurses themselves, through advocacy and solidarity, must continue to push the profession toward equity.

Racial Disparities in Patient Care

Racial disparities in patient care are among the most visible and well-documented manifestations of systemic racism in healthcare (Institute of Medicine 2003; Bailey et al. 2017). Despite advances in medicine, nursing science, and public health, people of color in the United States continue to face profound inequities in access to care, quality of treatment, and health outcomes. These disparities are not random variations but the result of historical oppression, structural inequities, implicit bias, and discriminatory practices that have become embedded in the healthcare system. For nurses who play a critical role in frontline care, understanding and addressing these inequities is essential to ensuring safe, ethical, and equitable care.

Research shows that even highly educated Black women with access to private healthcare are at significantly greater risk than their White counterparts (CDC 2017; Bailey et al. 2017). These disparities stem not from individual health behaviors but from structural racism, implicit bias in clinical decision-making, and a healthcare system that often fails to listen to and believe Black women when they report symptoms. Nurses working in obstetrics and maternal health are uniquely positioned to address these inequities, yet they too must confront the reality that standard practices often reinforce systemic biases.

Disparities also appear in pain management (Institute of Medicine 2003; Blair et al. 2011). Studies consistently reveal that Black and Hispanic patients are less likely to receive adequate pain assessment and treatment compared to White patients. Some providers continue to hold false beliefs about biological differences, such as the myth that Black patients have higher pain tolerance. These biases lead to under-prescribing of pain medication and dismissive treatment of patient concerns. For nurses, who are often responsible for initial pain assessments and advocacy, this inequity is especially critical. When nurses fail to challenge assumptions or advocate for patients, disparities in pain management are perpetuated.

Misdiagnosis and delayed treatment are further consequences of racial inequities in care (Institute of Medicine 2003; Bailey et al. 2017). Diagnostic overshadowing, in which a patient's symptoms are attributed to stereotypes rather than clinical evidence, disproportionately affects patients of color. For instance, Black patients with chest pain are less likely than White patients to receive prompt evaluation for cardiac conditions, even when presenting with identical symptoms. Indigenous patients presenting with mental health concerns may have their distress dismissed as substance use, reflecting stereotypes rather than evidence-based practice. Such disparities contribute directly to preventable morbidity and mortality and erode trust in the healthcare system.

The COVID-19 pandemic, for example, made these inequities painfully visible recently (CDC 2021; Bailey et al. 2017). Communities of color faced significantly higher rates of infection, hospitalization, and death compared to White populations. Inequities in testing access, triage decisions, and treatment reflected systemic racism. Many patients of color reported that their symptoms were minimized or that they were sent home from emergency departments only to later require critical care. Nurses on the frontlines of the pandemic witnessed how racial disparities, long documented in public health literature, translated into devastating outcomes during a global crisis.

Beyond acute care, disparities persist in preventive health services (National Academies of Sciences, Engineering, and Medicine 2019; CDC 2017). Black, Hispanic, and Indigenous populations are less likely to receive routine screenings such as mammograms, Pap smears, and colonoscopies. Language barriers, insurance status, provider bias, and inaccessible facilities all contribute to these gaps. The result is higher rates of late-stage cancer diagnoses and worse prognoses. Nurses, particularly those in primary care and community health, play a vital role in promoting screenings and preventive care, yet systemic barriers often undermine these efforts.

Another area of concern is mental health care (Williams and Mohammed 2013; Cuevas et al. 2019). Patients of color frequently encounter stigma, limited access to culturally competent providers, and inadequate treatment. Black men, for example, are disproportionately diagnosed with schizophrenia compared to White patients with similar symptoms, while mood disorders are often underdiagnosed. This reflects both implicit bias and cultural misunderstandings that shape diagnostic practices. Similarly, immigrant and refugee populations face challenges accessing mental health care due to language barriers, cultural stigma, and lack of insurance. Nurses trained in cultural humility can help bridge these gaps, but broader systemic reforms are needed to ensure equitable access.

Pediatric care also illustrates racial disparities (National Academies of Sciences, Engineering, and Medicine 2019; Bailey et al. 2017). Children of color are less likely to receive early interventions for developmental delays, less likely to be diagnosed with autism in a timely manner, and more likely to face disciplinary action in school settings for behaviors linked to unmet health needs. Nurses working in pediatrics and school health must confront the ways bias and structural inequities affect children's health trajectories from an early age. Addressing disparities in childhood care is particularly critical, as early health inequities often compound into lifelong disadvantages.

Across all of these examples, a common thread emerges: patients of color often experience not only poorer outcomes but also lower levels of respect, trust, and communication in their healthcare encounters (Cuevas et al. 2019; Institute of Medicine 2003). Many report feeling dismissed, unheard, or treated as less deserving of care. These experiences are not incidental but reflect the persistence of systemic racism in healthcare delivery. For nurses, who are consistently ranked among the most trusted professionals, addressing these inequities requires moving beyond technical competence to embrace advocacy, equity, and justice as core aspects of professional practice.

The persistence of racial disparities in patient care makes clear that inequities are not the result of isolated incidents but systemic issues that require structural change (Bailey et al. 2017; Yearby 2020). Nurses have a responsibility to identify and challenge these inequities, both in their individual practice and within the systems they work. This involves recognizing bias, advocating for patients, ensuring accessibility, and engaging in efforts to reform the policies and structures that perpetuate inequities. Only by confronting the realities of racial disparities in patient care can the nursing profession fulfill its ethical commitment to health equity.

Systemic and Structural Racism in Healthcare

While racial disparities in health outcomes and patient care are visible at the individual level, their roots lie in the broader structures of society and healthcare systems (Bailey et al. 2017; Yearby 2020). Systemic racism refers to the policies, practices, and institutional norms that perpetuate racial inequities, often without overt intent or explicit prejudice. For nurses, who work within these systems, it is crucial to recognize how structural racism shapes not only patient outcomes but also professional opportunities and workplace culture. Without addressing the systemic foundations of inequity, individual interventions risk being superficial or short-lived.

One of the most enduring legacies of systemic racism in healthcare is the impact of residential segregation and redlining (Yearby 2020; Bailey et al. 2017). For much of the twentieth century, discriminatory housing policies relegated Black, Indigenous, and other minority populations to under-resourced neighborhoods, often with limited access to healthcare facilities, grocery stores, safe housing, and green spaces. These social determinants of health have direct and lasting consequences. Communities subject to disinvestment and environmental hazards face higher rates of chronic illness, poorer mental health outcomes, and reduced life expectancy. Nurses practicing in these areas witness firsthand how geography shaped by racist policies translates into unequal health outcomes.

Structural racism is also embedded in the financing of healthcare (Yearby 2020; Bailey et al. 2017). Insurance coverage, which dictates access to care in the United States, is closely tied to employment. Because people of color are disproportionately represented in low-wage or unstable jobs that do not provide insurance, they are more likely to be uninsured or underinsured. Even when insured, minority populations often face higher deductibles or limited provider networks. Medicaid, which covers a disproportionate number of Black, Hispanic, and Indigenous patients, is underfunded compared to private insurance, leading to systemic inequities in resource allocation. For nurses, these disparities become visible when patients delay care, decline tests or medications due to cost, or are discharged without the supports needed for recovery.

Racism also operates within the design and use of clinical algorithms (Bailey et al. 2017; Yearby 2020). Recent studies have shown that widely used algorithms in healthcare incorporate racial "adjustments" that disadvantage patients of color. For example, estimated glomerular filtration rate (eGFR), a measure used to assess kidney function, historically included a "correction" for Black patients that assumed higher muscle mass. This adjustment artificially inflated kidney function estimates for Black patients, delaying referrals for transplant or specialty care. Similar adjustments in pulmonary function tests and obstetric risk scores have contributed to inequitable treatment decisions. Nurses, who rely on these algorithms in their practice, may inadvertently participate in systemic bias without realizing its impact. Recognizing and challenging such practices is an essential component of anti-racist nursing.

In nursing education, structural racism manifests in both curricula and institutional culture (National Academies of Sciences, Engineering, and Medicine 2019; Bailey et al. 2017). Textbooks often underrepresent the health concerns of minority populations or present them through a deficit-based lens. Case studies may default to White patients as the "norm," marginalizing the experiences of patients of color. Faculty diversity remains limited, and students of color frequently report experiencing bias, stereotyping, and lack of support. These inequities discourage retention and advancement, perpetuating the underrepresentation of minority nurses in the profession. Structural barriers such as standardized testing requirements, which may disadvantage students from marginalized backgrounds, further limit access to nursing education. Addressing these inequities requires curricular reform, faculty diversification, and institutional accountability in recruitment and retention.

Workplace culture also reflects systemic racism (Cuevas et al. 2019; Bailey et al. 2017). Nurses of color often describe environments where they are excluded from decision-making, overlooked for leadership opportunities, or subjected to microaggressions from colleagues and patients. These experiences are not isolated incidents but indicators of organizational structures that fail to support equity. When complaints of discrimination are minimized or dismissed, institutions reinforce a culture of silence and complicity. The psychological toll of such environments contributes to burnout and turnover among minority nurses, exacerbating workforce disparities.

Professional organizations and licensure bodies also play a role in perpetuating inequities (American Nurses Association 2015; Bailey et al. 2017). Minority nurses remain underrepresented in leadership positions within national associations, limiting their influence on policy and practice standards. Research funding continues to favor topics and methodologies that center White populations, leaving the health concerns of communities of color underexplored. Even efforts at diversity and inclusion can become tokenistic if they do not address systemic barriers and redistribute power. For nursing to move toward equity, professional structures must actively dismantle racism within their own ranks.

The cumulative impact of systemic racism is evident in the persistence of racial health disparities across generations (Williams and Mohammed 2013; Yearby 2020). These disparities are not explained by genetics or personal choices but by the unequal distribution of resources, opportunities, and respect. Nurses, positioned at the intersection of healthcare and community, are uniquely equipped to identify these systemic injustices and advocate for change. However, doing so requires moving beyond the individual encounter to interrogate the policies, practices, and structures that shape health.

Structural racism in healthcare is not an abstract concept but a daily reality that determines who receives care, how care is delivered, and whose voices are heard (Bailey et al. 2017; Yearby 2020). By naming and challenging these systemic inequities, nursing can begin to fulfill its ethical obligation to promote justice. This requires courage, persistence, and a willingness to confront uncomfortable truths, but the cost of inaction is the perpetuation of inequities that undermine both patients and the profession itself.

Toward Equity in Nursing Practice

If racial disparities are to be dismantled, nursing must move from acknowledgment to sustained action (American Nurses Association 2015; Bailey et al. 2017). Awareness of inequities is essential, but without systemic change, disparities will persist across generations. Advancing racial equity requires transformation at multiple levels: the bedside, the classroom, the workplace, and the policy arena. Nurses, as the largest segment of the healthcare workforce and the most trusted profession in the United States, hold enormous power to lead this transformation.

A first step toward equity involves cultivating anti-racist practice (Bailey et al. 2017; American Nurses Association 2015). This goes beyond cultural competence, which often reduces patient interactions to learning about "other" groups, to embrace cultural humility, which emphasizes lifelong reflection, openness to feedback, and recognition of power imbalances in care. Nurses must recognize their own biases, examine how these shape interactions with patients, and commit to dismantling them. This is not a one-time training but an ongoing professional responsibility. For example, when a Black patient reports pain, the nurse must consciously resist implicit stereotypes that might otherwise minimize or dismiss the concern, instead ensuring a thorough assessment and advocacy for appropriate treatment.

Nursing education must also be restructured to support equity (National Academies of Sciences, Engineering, and Medicine 2019; Bailey et al. 2017). Schools of nursing play a central role in shaping professional values and competencies, yet curricula have historically reflected Eurocentric perspectives and deficit-based views of minority populations. Reforms should include integrating the history of racism in healthcare, highlighting contributions of nurses of color, and teaching students how to identify and challenge structural inequities. Faculty diversity must also be prioritized, ensuring that students learn from and are mentored by leaders who reflect the diversity of the communities they will serve. Pipeline programs that support students of color in entering and completing nursing programs are essential, as are scholarships and financial supports that address barriers rooted in socioeconomic inequities.

Workplace environments must be transformed into spaces where nurses of color can thrive (Cuevas et al. 2019; Bailey et al. 2017). Institutions must adopt zero-tolerance policies for racism and discrimination, with clear reporting mechanisms and accountability structures. Support systems, such as affinity groups, mentorship programs, and leadership development initiatives, can help nurses of color feel included and valued. Pay equity audits and transparent promotion processes are essential for addressing structural inequities. Leadership positions must be opened to and actively filled by nurses of color, whose perspectives are critical to shaping policy, practice, and organizational culture. Without representation at decision-making tables, efforts toward equity will remain incomplete.

Policy advocacy is another vital component of advancing racial equity (American Nurses Association 2015; Yearby 2020). Nurses have long been active in shaping health policy, and racial equity must be central to these efforts. This includes advocating for equitable distribution of healthcare resources, supporting Medicaid expansion and other policies that reduce insurance gaps, and pressing for stronger enforcement of civil rights protections in healthcare. Nursing organizations can play a leadership role by issuing position statements on racism, lobbying for legislative change, and holding institutions accountable for equity outcomes.

Community engagement represents another avenue for nurses to advance equity (National Academies of Sciences, Engineering, and Medicine 2019; American Nurses Association 2015). Nurses often serve as bridges between healthcare systems and the communities they serve. By partnering with community organizations, churches, schools, and advocacy groups, nurses can help design interventions that are responsive to local needs and rooted in trust. Community-based participatory research, which positions community members as equal partners, provides a model for ensuring that interventions reflect the lived experiences of those most affected by inequities.

Technology and innovation must also be examined through an equity lens (Yearby 2020; Bailey et al. 2017). Electronic health records, telehealth platforms, and predictive algorithms can either reduce or exacerbate disparities depending on how they are designed and implemented. Nurses must advocate for inclusive technology that accounts for diverse populations, provides equitable access, and avoids embedding racial biases in data-driven tools.

Finally, the profession must embrace accountability (American Nurses Association 2015; Bailey et al. 2017). It is not enough to declare a commitment to diversity, equity, and inclusion; progress must be measured and reported. Institutions can track disparities in patient outcomes, workforce diversity, pay equity, and leadership representation, using these data to guide interventions and evaluate effectiveness. Nurses at all levels must demand transparency and hold themselves and their organizations accountable for advancing equity.

Toward equity in nursing practice means reimagining the profession itself (American Nurses Association 2015; Bailey et al. 2017). It requires confronting the ways in which racism has shaped healthcare historically and continues to shape it today. It requires equipping nurses with the tools, knowledge, and support to dismantle inequities, advocate for justice, and provide care that honors the dignity of every patient. While the task is daunting, it is also an opportunity for nursing to live out its most fundamental values, compassion, respect, and advocacy, by committing to a future where equity is not an aspiration but a reality.

Conclusion

Racial disparities in nursing are not incidental, nor are they confined to isolated events of prejudice (Bailey et al. 2017; Williams and Mohammed 2013). They are structural, systemic, and enduring, woven into the history of healthcare and the ongoing operations of its institutions. Throughout this chapter, the evidence has shown that inequities exist at every level of the nursing profession and the broader healthcare system from the underrepresentation and marginalization of nurses of color, to the unequal treatment and poorer health outcomes experienced by patients of color, to the policies and structures that perpetuate inequity. These realities demand that nursing as a profession confront racism not as a peripheral issue but as a central challenge to its ethical commitments and mission.

The analysis began by grounding racial disparities in their historical context (Smedley et al. 2003; Jones 2000). Legacies of slavery, segregation, and medical exploitation have left deep scars on communities of color and established patterns of mistrust that persist today. Within nursing, the exclusion of minority students and professionals created structural barriers that continue to shape representation and leadership. Understanding this history is essential because it demonstrates that racial disparities are not accidents of the present but the products of deliberate systems of exclusion and inequity.

The workforce dimension highlighted how nurses of color continue to face barriers in education, employment, and advancement (National Academies of Sciences, Engineering, and Medicine 2019; Bailey et al. 2017). Discrimination, pay inequities, microaggressions, and limited representation in leadership are not only unjust but also harmful to the profession as a whole. A diverse and inclusive workforce enhances patient care, improves cultural responsiveness, and strengthens the ability of nursing to serve an increasingly diverse population. Yet such diversity cannot be achieved without dismantling the structures that prevent minority nurses from entering, thriving, and leading within the profession.

Disparities in patient care make the consequences of systemic racism particularly stark (Institute of Medicine 2003; Bailey et al. 2017). Higher maternal mortality among Black women, inequities in pain management, misdiagnosis and delayed treatment, and disparities in preventive care and mental health services demonstrate how bias and systemic barriers translate directly into preventable suffering and death. Nurses, who play a frontline role in patient care, are uniquely positioned to intervene, advocate, and ensure that all patients receive equitable treatment. But this requires conscious effort to recognize bias, resist paternalism, and embrace partnership with patients as equal participants in their care.

At the structural level, racism is embedded in housing policies, insurance systems, clinical algorithms, educational curricula, and organizational culture (Yearby 2020; Bailey et al. 2017). These systemic factors create and perpetuate inequities across generations. Nurses must therefore move beyond individual practice to engage in systemic advocacy pushing for reforms that expand access, ensure accountability, and redistribute resources to achieve equity. Professional organizations, educational institutions, and policymakers all have a role to play in dismantling the structures that produce and sustain racial inequities.

The way forward lies in embracing anti-racist nursing practice, which includes cultural humility, educational reform, workforce diversity, leadership representation, and policy advocacy (American Nurses Association 2015; Bailey et al. 2017). Anti-racism requires continuous reflection, courage to confront uncomfortable truths, and commitment to dismantling unjust structures. It is not a one-time initiative but a lifelong professional responsibility. By embracing anti-racist practice, nursing can move closer to fulfilling its promise of holistic, compassionate, and just care for all.

In conclusion, addressing racial disparities is not an additional task layered onto nursing practice; it is integral to the profession's mission (American Nurses Association 2015). Nurses are trusted advocates, caregivers, and leaders. With this trust comes the responsibility to challenge injustice wherever it appears, whether in the classroom, the clinic, the boardroom, or the community. The profession cannot claim to uphold human dignity or promote health equity if it remains complicit in structures that perpetuate racial inequities. By committing to equity and justice, nursing can lead healthcare toward a more inclusive future, one where race no longer predicts the quality of care or the outcomes of health.

References

American Nurses Association. Code of ethics for nurses with interpretive statements. ANA; 2015.

Bailey ZD, Krieger N, Agénor M, Graves J, Linos N, Bassett MT. Structural racism and health inequities in the USA: evidence and interventions. Lancet. 2017;389(10077):1453–63. https://doi.org/10.1016/S0140-6736(17)30569-X.

Blair IV, Steiner JF, Havranek EP. Unconscious (implicit) bias and health disparities: where do we go from here? Perm J. 2011;15(2):71–8. https://doi.org/10.7812/TPP/11-018.

Centers for Disease Control and Prevention. African American health: creating equal opportunities for health. 2017. https://www.cdc.gov/vitalsigns/aahealth/index.html.

Centers for Disease Control and Prevention. COVID-19 racial and ethnic health disparities. 2021. https://www.cdc.gov/coronavirus/2019-ncov/community/health-equity/racial-ethnic-disparities/index.html.

Cuevas AG, O'Brien K, Saha S. African American experiences in healthcare: "I always feel like I'm getting skipped over". Health Serv Res. 2019;54(2):462–76. https://doi.org/10.1111/1475-6773.13111.

Institute of Medicine. Unequal treatment: confronting racial and ethnic disparities in health care. National Academies Press; 2003.

Jones CP. Levels of racism: A theoretic framework and a gardener's tale. Am J Public Health. 2000;90(8):1212–5. https://doi.org/10.2105/AJPH.90.8.1212.

National Academies of Sciences, Engineering, and Medicine. Integrating social care into the delivery of health care: moving upstream to improve the nation's health. National Academies Press; 2019.

Smedley, B. D., Stith, A. Y., & Nelson, A. R. (Eds.). (2003). Unequal treatment: confronting racial and ethnic disparities in health care. National Academies Press.

Williams DR, Mohammed SA. Racism and health I: pathways and scientific evidence. Am Behav Sci. 2013;57(8):1152–73. https://doi.org/10.1177/0002764213487340.

Yearby R. Structural racism and health disparities: reconfiguring the social determinants of health framework to include the root cause. J Law Med Ethics. 2020;48(3):518–26. https://doi.org/10.1177/1073110520958876.

Part II

Systemic Inequities and Contemporary Challenges

Gender Equity and Discrimination 4

Introduction to Gender Equity in Nursing

The concept of gender equity is central to understanding both the history and the future of nursing (World Health Organization 2019; American Nurses Association 2015). Equity, distinct from equality, recognizes that individuals may require different resources, opportunities, and supports in order to achieve fair outcomes. While equality implies sameness, equity demands responsiveness to structural barriers and systemic disadvantages. In the context of nursing, gender equity refers to ensuring that nurses of all genders have equal opportunities for education, advancement, recognition, and compensation, while patients of all genders receive care that is unbiased, respectful, and tailored to their specific needs. Despite progress in recent decades, gender inequities remain pervasive in healthcare, shaping both professional practice and patient outcomes.

Nursing, as a profession, has long been entwined with gendered expectations (Carroll and Riska 2002; World Health Organization 2019). Since the days of Florence Nightingale, nursing has been framed as a "calling" associated with feminine ideals of selflessness, nurturing, and caregiving. These cultural associations elevated the moral reputation of nursing but also constrained it, reinforcing stereotypes that nursing was "women's work" and positioning it in a subordinate relationship to medicine, a field historically dominated by men. Such dynamics have had lasting consequences for the profession's status, autonomy, and compensation. Even today, nursing salaries lag behind comparable professions, a disparity that cannot be understood apart from the broader context of gendered labor devaluation.

At the same time, gender inequities within nursing are not limited to women's disadvantage (World Health Organization 2019; Carroll and Riska 2002). While women represent the overwhelming majority of the nursing workforce, men in nursing often confront their own challenges. They may face stigma for entering a "feminized" profession, encounter assumptions that they are less caring or nurturing, or be stereotyped into roles perceived as requiring physical strength, such as

N. Nami, *Unraveling Social Justice Issues in Nursing*,
https://doi.org/10.1007/978-3-032-26512-8_4

emergency or intensive care units. Male nurses are sometimes pushed more quickly into leadership roles, reflecting the persistence of a "glass escalator" effect in which men are advantaged in female-dominated professions. These dynamics illustrate that gender inequity in nursing is complex, affecting individuals differently depending on context, role, and identity.

The patient side of healthcare also reflects gender inequities (Institute of Medicine 2001; Vermeulen and Luyten 2018). Women's health concerns have historically been neglected, trivialized, or misunderstood within medicine. For decades, women were excluded from clinical trials, leading to treatment protocols based primarily on male physiology and creating blind spots in diagnosis and care. For example, heart disease in women often presents with different symptoms than in men, yet diagnostic tools and clinical training long emphasized male-centered presentations, resulting in delayed diagnoses and worse outcomes for women. Similarly, pain experienced by women is more likely to be dismissed or attributed to psychological causes, reflecting both implicit bias and longstanding gender stereotypes.

Gender equity in healthcare is also inseparable from intersectionality (Celis et al. 2013; World Health Organization 2019). Gender does not operate in isolation but interacts with race, class, sexuality, and disability to produce layered inequities. For instance, while maternal mortality disproportionately affects women, Black women in the United States face mortality rates that are three to four times higher than those of White women. Such disparities cannot be explained by gender alone but by the interplay of racism and sexism in both healthcare delivery and society at large. Intersectionality reminds us that gender equity cannot be achieved without attention to the multiple systems of oppression that shape people's experiences.

The professional and ethical commitments of nursing demand engagement with gender equity (American Nurses Association 2015). The American Nurses Association Code of Ethics emphasizes justice, respect for human dignity, and advocacy for vulnerable populations. Nurses, who often serve as patients' first point of contact and primary advocates within healthcare systems, are uniquely positioned to recognize and address gendered inequities in care. Yet this requires more than individual awareness; it demands systemic changes in education, practice, policy, and organizational culture.

Historically, efforts to promote gender equity in nursing and healthcare have made important strides, from Title IX legislation that expanded educational opportunities to growing advocacy for equal pay and family leave policies (American Association of University Women 2021; National Women's Law Center 2020). Nevertheless, inequities remain entrenched, with persistent pay gaps, underrepresentation of women in healthcare leadership, barriers for men in nursing, and ongoing gender bias in patient care. These inequities not only harm individuals but also undermine the effectiveness and integrity of healthcare systems.

This chapter will examine gender equity and discrimination in nursing through multiple lenses. It will begin by analyzing gender disparities within the nursing profession, including pay inequities, leadership gaps, and workplace discrimination (American Association of University Women 2021; Kalaitzi et al. 2017). It will then turn to patient care, exploring how gender bias shapes diagnosis, treatment, and outcomes for women, men, and nonbinary individuals. The discussion will extend to systemic and structural forms of gender discrimination in healthcare, such as institutional policies, research practices, and cultural expectations of caregiving. Finally, the chapter will explore pathways toward equity, highlighting strategies for reform in nursing education, clinical practice, workplace policies, and health advocacy.

The introduction of this chapter sets the stage for a critical examination of how gender inequities remain embedded in nursing and healthcare, despite progress toward equality (World Health Organization 2019; Stamarski and Son Hing 2015). By framing gender equity as both a professional responsibility and a moral imperative, this chapter emphasizes the urgency of dismantling gender discrimination in all its forms. Nurses, as trusted professionals and frontline advocates, must lead this effort not only for the sake of fairness within their own profession but also to ensure that patients of all genders receive the care they deserve.

Gender Disparities Within the Nursing Profession

Although nursing has historically been and continues to be a female-dominated profession, gender disparities remain embedded in its structures, culture, and practices (World Health Organization 2019; Carroll and Riska 2002). The assumption that women "naturally" belong in nursing has both elevated the profession's image as nurturing and compassionate and simultaneously devalued its status as skilled, intellectual, and autonomous work. This paradox continues to shape how nurses are compensated, how they are represented in leadership, and how they are perceived both inside and outside the healthcare system.

One of the most visible forms of gender inequity in nursing is the persistence of pay gaps (American Association of University Women 2021; National Women's Law Center 2020). Research consistently demonstrates that male nurses earn higher salaries than their female counterparts, even when controlling for role, years of experience, and educational attainment. The "glass escalator" effect where men in female-dominated professions advance more quickly to higher-paying or supervisory roles remains evident in nursing. Men are disproportionately represented in administrative or leadership positions relative to their numbers in the profession, and this creates a structural imbalance. Women, despite representing nearly 90% of the workforce, are more likely to be concentrated in bedside and support roles that are undervalued financially and professionally. The pay gap is not simply a matter of personal salary; it reflects broader patterns of gendered devaluation of labor and undermines the economic security of a largely female workforce.

Leadership disparities further reveal how gender shapes opportunities in nursing (Kalaitzi et al. 2017; Carnes and Bland 2007). While women dominate the profession numerically, they remain underrepresented in positions of power within healthcare institutions, academia, and professional organizations. Deanships of nursing schools, chief nursing officer roles, and national policy boards are still disproportionately held by men or by a relatively small subset of women who overcome systemic barriers. These barriers include implicit bias, structural discrimination, and lack of mentorship opportunities. Leadership inequities also emerge in the intersection of nursing with medicine; while medicine is more gender-balanced than in past decades, men continue to dominate the highest-paying specialties and hospital executive roles, leaving nursing disproportionately influenced by male-dominated hierarchies.

Discrimination and stereotyping also persist in subtle and overt ways (Stamarski and Son Hing 2015; Moss-Racusin et al. 2012). Women in nursing leadership often confront the "double bind" of being judged as too passive if they conform to gender norms or too aggressive if they assert authority. Men in nursing encounter different stereotypes, often being questioned about their masculinity or assumed to be better suited for technical, emergency, or physically demanding areas of practice. Some male nurses are steered away from specialties like pediatrics or obstetrics, reflecting ongoing assumptions that caregiving roles in those areas are inherently female. These stereotypes create professional silos that restrict opportunity, perpetuate bias, and undermine the idea that nursing is a profession grounded in skill rather than gendered identity.

Workplace harassment and discrimination are also realities for many nurses (Stamarski and Son Hing 2015; World Health Organization 2019). Women in healthcare frequently report experiencing sexual harassment from colleagues, supervisors, or patients, and these experiences can affect their career progression and mental health. Men in nursing, while less likely to experience sexual harassment, may face verbal abuse or discrimination rooted in gender stereotypes. In both cases, inadequate institutional responses to harassment perpetuate cultures of silence and fear, undermining professional equity and workplace safety.

The gender inequities within nursing cannot be understood in isolation from broader social and cultural norms (Heggeness and Murray-Close 2019; Carroll and Riska 2002). The caregiving work historically assigned to women has long been undervalued both economically and socially. Nursing salaries lag behind those of professions requiring similar levels of education and responsibility, not because of the intrinsic value of the work but because of its association with women. This "wage penalty" for female-dominated professions is well-documented across industries and reinforces structural inequities in nursing. Men's higher pay and accelerated advancement within nursing do not contradict this trend; rather, they highlight the gendered dynamics by which men are rewarded for entering "women's work" while women as a group continue to face systemic disadvantage.

Addressing gender disparities in nursing requires more than acknowledging them (American Nurses Association 2015; World Health Organization 2019). It demands structural change in how nursing education, leadership, and workplace policies are designed. Mentorship programs for women and men alike must challenge stereotypes and create equitable opportunities for advancement. Pay transparency and policy reforms are needed to close wage gaps. Institutional cultures must evolve to eliminate harassment and discrimination and to promote inclusivity. These changes are not simply about fairness to nurses themselves; they are essential for the integrity and sustainability of the profession. A workforce that is equitably compensated, free from discrimination, and representative of diverse leadership is better positioned to deliver high-quality, equitable patient care.

In sum, gender disparities within nursing reveal the contradictions of a profession that is both overwhelmingly female and yet still subject to the forces of gender inequity (World Health Organization 2019; Heggeness and Murray-Close 2019). The persistence of pay gaps, leadership imbalances, stereotypes, and harassment demonstrates that gender equity has not yet been achieved. Nurses must confront these inequities not only for their own professional advancement but also to ensure that nursing as a whole continues to grow as a respected, just, and inclusive profession.

Gender Disparities in Patient Care

While gender inequities within the nursing profession shape the opportunities and experiences of nurses themselves, inequities in patient care reflect how deeply gender bias permeates healthcare delivery (Institute of Medicine 2001; Vermeulen and Luyten 2018). Patients do not enter healthcare systems as blank slates; they carry with them histories, social roles, and identities that influence how they are perceived and treated by clinicians. The interaction between patient identity and provider bias whether conscious or unconscious produces patterns of discrimination that undermine the principles of equity, justice, and dignity that healthcare professions, including nursing, are ethically bound to uphold.

Women's health disparities are perhaps the most visible example of gender bias in patient care (Institute of Medicine 2001; Johnson et al. 2020). Historically, medical research and clinical education were built on the assumption of the male body as the norm. For decades, women were excluded from clinical trials under the rationale that hormonal fluctuations complicated research results or that including women of childbearing age posed liability risks. As a result, diagnostic standards, drug dosages, and treatment guidelines were largely developed based on male physiology. This systemic exclusion has had profound consequences. Conditions such as cardiovascular disease, which remains the leading cause of death for women in the United States, often present differently in women than in men. Women are more likely to experience non-classic symptoms such as fatigue, shortness of breath, or nausea rather than the stereotypical chest pain emphasized in medical training. Consequently, women are more likely to be misdiagnosed or to experience delays in receiving life-saving interventions such as angioplasty.

Pain management also reflects entrenched gender disparities (Vermeulen and Luyten 2018; Johnson et al. 2020). Studies consistently show that women's reports of pain are taken less seriously than men's, with healthcare providers more likely to attribute women's symptoms to psychological causes such as anxiety or depression. Women are also more likely to be prescribed sedatives rather than analgesics, reinforcing stereotypes that they are "emotional" rather than experiencing genuine physiological suffering. This bias has life-altering consequences, as untreated or undertreated pain can lead to chronic disability, diminished quality of life, and erosion of trust in healthcare systems. Nurses, who often serve as patients' first advocates, are uniquely positioned to challenge such disparities by validating patients' experiences, advocating for appropriate interventions, and resisting the temptation to minimize symptoms based on gendered assumptions.

Reproductive health provides another lens through which to understand gender inequities in patient care (Bick and Chang 2021; World Health Organization 2019). Access to contraception, abortion, prenatal care, and maternal health services remains uneven, shaped by both systemic policies and provider-level biases. Maternal mortality in the United States particularly among Black women stands as a stark indicator of gendered and racialized inequities. Despite advances in obstetric medicine, women in the United States are more likely to die in childbirth than women in other high-income nations. These outcomes cannot be explained solely by socioeconomic status or comorbidities; rather, they reflect cumulative effects of racism, sexism, and structural neglect within healthcare systems. Nurses in obstetric, gynecologic, and neonatal care must therefore be especially attentive to how gender and race intersect to shape maternal and infant outcomes.

Gender inequities are not confined to women (Baker et al. 2014; Celis et al. 2013). Men, too, face specific disparities in healthcare. Cultural norms around masculinity often discourage men from seeking preventive care or acknowledging health concerns, leading to delayed diagnoses and poorer outcomes in conditions such as mental illness, cardiovascular disease, and certain cancers. Depression and anxiety in men may be underdiagnosed because they present with irritability, anger, or risk-taking behaviors rather than the "classic" symptoms more readily associated with women. Similarly, men are more likely to die by suicide, yet less likely to seek or receive mental health treatment. Nurses who work in primary care, emergency departments, and mental health settings must be equipped to recognize these patterns and challenge the gendered assumptions that contribute to them.

Beyond the binary categories of men and women, healthcare systems are increasingly challenged to address the inequities faced by transgender and nonbinary patients (Celis et al. 2013; World Health Organization 2019). These individuals encounter widespread discrimination, ranging from refusal of care to inappropriate curiosity about their bodies to a lack of providers trained in gender-affirming practices. Transgender patients may avoid healthcare settings altogether for fear of stigma, leading to unmet health needs and preventable complications. Nursing, with its emphasis on holistic and person-centered care, has both an ethical obligation and an opportunity to lead in creating inclusive environments for patients across the gender spectrum. This includes ensuring access to appropriate documentation, respecting chosen names and pronouns, and advocating for policies that protect transgender patients from discrimination.

Intersectionality is critical to understanding how gender disparities manifest in patient care (Celis et al. 2013; Bick and Chang 2021). Women of color, low-income women, immigrant women, and disabled women often face compounded disadvantages that amplify inequities. For example, an immigrant woman with limited English proficiency may experience delays in maternal care not only because of gender bias but also because of linguistic and cultural barriers. A disabled woman may be denied access to reproductive health services because of assumptions about her sexual activity or reproductive capacity. Similarly, men of color may be less likely to receive pain management than White men, reflecting racial as well as gender bias. Intersectionality underscores that gender cannot be disentangled from other axes of inequality and that nursing practice must be attentive to these overlapping forms of oppression.

Addressing gender disparities in patient care requires a multipronged approach (American Nurses Association 2015; Vermeulen and Luyten 2018). Nurses must cultivate self-awareness of their own biases, advocate for inclusive policies, and ensure that patients' voices are central to decision-making processes. Equitable care is not achieved by treating everyone the same but by responding to the unique needs and contexts of each patient. This means recognizing that a woman's complaint of chest pain may require different diagnostic consideration than a man's, or that a transgender patient's refusal of care may reflect prior traumatic experiences rather than "noncompliance". Ultimately, nursing's commitment to advocacy and holistic care positions it as a powerful force in challenging gender bias in patient care and promoting health equity for all.

Systemic and Structural Gender Discrimination in Healthcare

Gender disparities in healthcare do not arise solely from individual bias or interpersonal interactions (Stamarski and Son Hing 2015; World Health Organization 2019). They are sustained and amplified by systemic and structural forces embedded within healthcare institutions, policies, and cultural norms. These structural inequities reflect longstanding patterns of exclusion, underrepresentation, and undervaluation of women's and gender-diverse people's needs. Understanding these broader dynamics is crucial for moving beyond isolated reforms toward comprehensive strategies for gender equity.

Historically, healthcare institutions and medical research have been organized around male-centered norms (Institute of Medicine 2001; National Academies of Sciences, Engineering, and Medicine 2018). Until the 1990s, women were routinely excluded from clinical trials, often justified by concerns about hormonal variability or potential pregnancy. This exclusion resulted in treatment standards that were based almost exclusively on male physiology, leaving women at risk of ineffective or even harmful care. The consequences of this systemic bias are evident today: women are more likely to experience adverse drug reactions, as dosages are often calibrated to male bodies, and diagnostic criteria for major illnesses such as cardiovascular disease still reflect male-centered symptom profiles. The absence of women's bodies and experiences in the construction of biomedical knowledge is not an accident but a structural form of discrimination that continues to undermine women's health outcomes.

Beyond research, policies and institutional structures also reinforce gender inequities (Stamarski and Son Hing 2015; World Health Organization 2019). Workplace policies around maternity leave, childcare support, and flexible scheduling often fail to meet the needs of female healthcare workers, many of whom shoulder disproportionate caregiving responsibilities. The lack of robust parental leave policies in the United States, for example, places particular strain on women in nursing, forcing them to return to work prematurely or risk losing career advancement opportunities. At the same time, men who seek parental leave may face stigma or professional penalties, reinforcing gendered expectations about caregiving roles. These policies reflect deeper structural assumptions about gender, work, and family that disadvantage both women and men in different ways.

Structural inequities also manifest in the unequal distribution of resources for gender-specific health needs (World Health Organization 2019; Bick and Chang 2021). Women's health services, particularly reproductive health, are chronically underfunded and politically contested, leading to reduced access and availability. Clinics offering abortion or comprehensive reproductive care are often targets of legislative restrictions, undermining the ability of women to exercise autonomy over their bodies. Meanwhile, men's health initiatives, such as prostate cancer awareness, have historically received more consistent funding and public attention, illustrating how societal values shape resource allocation in gendered ways. For transgender and nonbinary individuals, systemic exclusion is even more pronounced, with many insurance plans refusing to cover gender-affirming care and many institutions lacking providers trained in affirming practices.

Another dimension of systemic gender discrimination is the cultural expectation of caregiving, which permeates both the nursing profession and healthcare delivery more broadly (Carroll and Riska 2002; Heggeness and Murray-Close 2019). Nursing's historical association with feminine qualities of nurturing and sacrifice has often been used to justify low wages and limited autonomy. This devaluation of caregiving as "women's work" extends into the healthcare system's reliance on unpaid or underpaid family caregivers, the majority of whom are women. These cultural and structural dynamics create a cycle in which caregiving labor is consistently undervalued, despite being essential to both individual health and the functioning of healthcare systems.

Institutional culture also reinforces gender inequities through subtle and overt practices (Stamarski and Son Hing 2015; Moss-Racusin et al. 2012). In academic medicine and healthcare leadership, men are often presumed to be natural leaders, while women face higher scrutiny and lower rates of promotion. Gender bias in performance evaluations, mentorship opportunities, and publication credit perpetuates inequalities in recognition and advancement. Harassment and discrimination within healthcare institutions further reinforce hostile environments that drive women and gender-diverse individuals out of leadership pathways. The problem is not individual "bad actors" alone but organizational cultures that tolerate or normalize inequitable treatment.

The structural nature of gender discrimination means that solutions must go beyond changing individual attitudes to transforming institutions and systems (Stamarski and Son Hing 2015; World Health Organization 2019). Addressing research bias requires enforcing policies that mandate gender diversity in clinical trials and ensuring that results are analyzed by sex and gender. Reforming workplace policies means not only expanding parental leave but also creating equitable systems of evaluation that recognize and accommodate caregiving responsibilities. Redistributing resources toward women's health and gender-affirming care requires challenging the political and cultural ideologies that render these services less worthy of investment. And transforming organizational culture requires deliberate strategies to dismantle hierarchies that privilege male leadership and devalue caregiving labor.

For nurses, recognizing the systemic nature of gender discrimination is particularly important (American Nurses Association 2015; World Health Organization 2019). While individual acts of compassion and advocacy are necessary, they are insufficient if the structures within which nurses work continue to produce inequity. Nurses must therefore engage at multiple levels bedside, organizational, and policy to advocate for changes that address the root causes of gender inequities. By situating gender discrimination within broader structural and systemic contexts, nursing can position itself as a leader in advancing equity not only for patients but also for the healthcare workforce as a whole.

Toward Gender Equity in Nursing and Healthcare

The persistence of gender inequities in both the nursing workforce and patient care underscores the urgent need for intentional and systemic reforms (World Health Organization 2019; Stamarski and Son Hing 2015). Achieving gender equity requires more than surface-level inclusion or symbolic gestures; it demands structural transformation, accountability, and cultural change. Nursing, as both a profession and a social force, holds a unique position to lead this transformation. Because nurses represent the largest segment of the healthcare workforce and hold a reputation for public trust, they are well positioned to advocate for gender equity in ways that can influence both professional practice and broader healthcare systems.

One crucial pathway toward equity is addressing wage disparities and advancing pay transparency (American Association of University Women 2021; National Women's Law Center 2020). The gender pay gap remains one of the most visible inequities in nursing, with women earning less than men despite representing the overwhelming majority of the workforce. Closing this gap requires policy reforms that mandate transparent reporting of salaries, enforce equal pay for equal work, and provide mechanisms for accountability within healthcare institutions. Pay transparency not only benefits individual nurses but also strengthens the profession by affirming the value of nursing labor as skilled, intellectual, and essential. By advocating for and implementing fair compensation structures, nursing leaders can begin to dismantle the historical devaluation of caregiving work.

Representation in leadership must also be a priority (Kalaitzi et al. 2017; Carnes and Bland 2007). Increasing gender diversity in leadership roles both within nursing itself and across broader healthcare administration is essential to dismantling hierarchical structures that privilege male voices. Nursing schools and healthcare organizations must intentionally mentor and promote women and gender-diverse professionals into decision-making positions. Leadership development programs that prioritize equity can help ensure that diverse perspectives shape institutional priorities, research agendas, and patient care strategies. Nurses in leadership roles are especially well positioned to challenge policies that perpetuate inequity, model inclusive practices, and drive cultural change.

Policy reforms are another essential tool for advancing gender equity (National Women's Law Center 2020; American Nurses Association 2015). Advocacy for comprehensive family leave policies, flexible scheduling, and institutional supports for caregivers is necessary to address systemic barriers faced by many nurses. Ensuring that both women and men can take parental leave without stigma or professional penalty helps to redistribute caregiving responsibilities more equitably and normalizes shared family roles. At the same time, expanding access to affordable childcare and supporting nursing parents in the workplace reduces the attrition of skilled professionals who might otherwise be forced to leave the field. Nurses, as advocates and constituents, have the power to push for legislative reforms that expand these protections beyond individual institutions to the healthcare sector as a whole.

Educational reform also plays a vital role in dismantling gender inequities (National Academies of Sciences, Engineering, and Medicine 2018; American Nurses Association 2015). Nursing curricula must address implicit bias, cultural humility, and the impact of gender on health outcomes. By embedding gender equity into the core of nursing education, future nurses will be better equipped to identify and challenge discriminatory practices in both patient care and professional contexts. Nursing education must also move beyond binary understandings of gender to prepare students to care for transgender and nonbinary patients, whose health needs are often ignored or marginalized. Integrating gender studies perspectives into nursing education ensures that new generations of nurses enter the profession with a more nuanced and justice-oriented approach to equity.

In clinical practice, adopting gender-sensitive approaches is critical for ensuring equitable patient outcomes (Vermeulen and Luyten 2018; Institute of Medicine 2001). Nurses must remain attentive to how gender shapes patients' experiences of illness, diagnosis, and treatment. This involves not only validating patient concerns but also advocating for care that is inclusive and responsive to diverse needs. For example, a nurse caring for a woman presenting with atypical chest pain must recognize the possibility of cardiovascular disease and advocate for appropriate diagnostic testing, even if prevailing norms suggest otherwise. Similarly, nurses must champion the inclusion of transgender patients in preventive care services, ensuring that gender identity does not become a barrier to routine screenings and interventions.

Research is another arena where nursing can advance gender equity (National Academies of Sciences, Engineering, and Medicine 2018; Johnson et al. 2020). Historically, women and gender-diverse individuals have been underrepresented in health research, resulting in evidence gaps that perpetuate inequities in care. Nursing research can help fill these gaps by focusing on the experiences of marginalized populations, evaluating the impact of gendered disparities, and developing interventions tailored to diverse needs. Moreover, promoting equity in research requires structural reforms, including funding priorities that explicitly value gender equity and peer review processes that recognize the importance of inclusive study design. Nurses engaged in research must not only generate new knowledge but also ensure that such knowledge informs clinical practice and policy.

Finally, advancing gender equity in nursing requires sustained advocacy and coalition-building (American Nurses Association 2015; World Health Organization 2019). Nurses must partner with other professionals, patients, and community organizations to push for systemic reforms. This includes advocating for equitable healthcare access, reproductive justice, and protections for transgender and nonbinary individuals. Nursing organizations such as the American Nurses Association and the International Council of Nurses have already begun incorporating equity into their agendas, but these efforts must be expanded and deepened. Nurses as individuals and as a collective must consistently raise their voices against inequity, whether in institutional decision-making, public policy debates, or community advocacy.

The path toward gender equity in nursing and healthcare is complex and requires a multifaceted strategy (Stamarski and Son Hing 2015; World Health Organization 2019). It involves dismantling structural inequities in pay and leadership, reforming workplace and family policies, transforming education and research, and fostering inclusive clinical practices. Most importantly, it requires cultural change challenging the deep-seated assumptions that undervalue caregiving, marginalize women's voices, and exclude gender-diverse individuals. By embracing this challenge, nursing can not only advance equity within its own profession but also contribute to broader social change. Gender equity in healthcare is not merely an aspirational goal; it is a necessary condition for ethical, effective, and just care.

Conclusion

Gender inequities in nursing and healthcare are neither incidental nor inevitable (Stamarski and Son Hing 2015; World Health Organization 2019). They are the result of historical patterns, structural arrangements, and cultural norms that continue to shape how nurses work, how patients are cared for, and how resources are distributed. This chapter has traced these inequities across multiple dimensions: the professional workforce, patient care, systemic structures, and the broader cultural landscape in which nursing operates. At every level, gender plays a critical role in producing advantages for some while constraining opportunities and outcomes for others.

Within the nursing profession, women have long faced barriers to equal pay, advancement, and recognition, despite comprising the vast majority of the workforce (American Association of University Women 2021; Kalaitzi et al. 2017). Men in nursing, while fewer in number, often experience the opposite dynamic an accelerated path to leadership roles and higher salaries, reflecting the persistence of the "glass escalator". These inequities illustrate the paradox of a profession both dominated by women and still shaped by structural gendered disadvantage. Addressing these issues requires dismantling entrenched hierarchies and affirming the inherent value of nursing as skilled labor deserving of equitable compensation and respect.

In patient care, gender inequities are just as pervasive (Institute of Medicine 2001; Vermeulen and Luyten 2018). Women continue to face delayed diagnoses, inadequate pain management, and higher risks in maternal and reproductive health. Men, meanwhile, encounter stigma that discourages preventive care and mental health treatment, while transgender and nonbinary patients remain marginalized and often excluded from basic healthcare access. Intersectionality further complicates these disparities, as gender interacts with race, class, and disability to produce compounded disadvantages. Nurses, with their commitment to advocacy and holistic care, are uniquely positioned to confront these inequities at the bedside and beyond.

At the systemic level, gender inequities are reinforced by research practices, institutional policies, and cultural expectations of caregiving (Institute of Medicine 2001; Heggeness and Murray-Close 2019). The historical exclusion of women from clinical trials, the chronic underfunding of women's health and reproductive services, and workplace policies that fail to support parental leave or caregiving responsibilities all demonstrate that inequity is not just interpersonal; it is built into the very structures of healthcare. These systemic forces require systemic solutions, including reforms to research protocols, policy changes in employment and benefits, and deliberate efforts to dismantle institutional cultures of bias and exclusion.

The path forward is clear: nursing must embrace a proactive commitment to gender equity (American Nurses Association 2015; World Health Organization 2019). This means advancing pay transparency, supporting diverse leadership, reforming education to address bias and inclusivity, expanding equitable family leave policies, and ensuring that research and practice are attentive to gender in all its forms. It also means recognizing that gender equity is inseparable from other struggles for justice, including racial equity, disability rights, and LGBTQ+ inclusivity. Nurses must see themselves not only as caregivers but also as advocates for systemic change.

Ultimately, gender equity is not simply about fairness within the profession or improved outcomes for specific patient groups (World Health Organization 2019; American Nurses Association 2015). It is about fulfilling nursing's ethical obligation to uphold human dignity, promote justice, and deliver holistic care. Equity strengthens the profession, enhances patient outcomes, and moves healthcare systems closer to their fundamental mission of serving all people without bias. As the most trusted professionals in healthcare, nurses have both the authority and the responsibility to lead this transformation.

The work of achieving gender equity is ongoing, requiring vigilance, courage, and collaboration (Stamarski and Son Hing 2015; Kalaitzi et al. 2017). It will not be accomplished through isolated reforms but through sustained commitment at every level from the classroom to the clinic to the halls of policy-making. By embracing this challenge, nursing can ensure that gender is no longer a determinant of professional opportunity or patient outcome. In doing so, the profession will not only honor its history of advocacy but also secure its role as a leader in the broader movement for health justice.

References

American Association of University Women. The simple truth about the gender pay gap. 2021. https://www.aauw.org/resources/research/simple-truth/.

American Nurses Association. Code of ethics for nurses with interpretive statements. ANA; 2015.

Baker P, Dworkin SL, Tong S, Banks I, Shand T, Yamey G. The men's health gap: men must be included in the global health equity agenda. BMJ. 2014;349:g4483. https://doi.org/10.1136/bmj.g4483.

Bick D, Chang YS. Maternal mortality in the United States: time to increase accountability for women's health. Int J Gynecol Obstet. 2021;154(2):401–3. https://doi.org/10.1002/ijgo.13641.

Carnes M, Bland C. Viewpoint: a challenge to academic health centers: women faculty in clinical and translational science. Acad Med. 2007;82(2):191–9. https://doi.org/10.1097/ACM.0b013e31802d9390.

Carroll L, Riska E. Medicine as a patriarchal system: the changing role of women in medicine. Rowman & Littlefield; 2002.

Celis, K., Kantola, J., Waylen, G., & Weldon, S. L. (Eds.). (2013). The Oxford handbook of gender and politics. Oxford University Press.

Heggeness ML, Murray-Close M. Gender and the rise of the care economy. Demography. 2019;56(5):1645–69. https://doi.org/10.1007/s13524-019-00786-w.

Institute of Medicine. Exploring the biological contributions to human health: does sex matter? National Academies Press; 2001.

Johnson PA, Fitzgerald T, Salganicoff A, editors. Sex-specific reporting of scientific research: a workshop summary. National Academies Press; 2020.

Kalaitzi S, Czabanowska K, Fowler-Davis S, Brand H, Iliopoulos E. Women, leadership and the health sector: barriers and facilitators. Int J Environ Res Public Health. 2017;14(7):683. https://doi.org/10.3390/ijerph14070683.

Moss-Racusin CA, Dovidio JF, Brescoll VL, Graham MJ, Handelsman J. Science faculty's subtle gender biases favor male students. Proc Natl Acad Sci. 2012;109(41):16474–9. https://doi.org/10.1073/pnas.1211286109.

National Academies of Sciences, Engineering, and Medicine. Sex- and gender-based analysis in health research: a roadmap for policy, practice, and research. National Academies Press; 2018.

National Women's Law Center. The wage gap: the who, how, why, and what to do. 2020. https://nwlc.org/resources/the-wage-gap-the-who-how-why-and-what-to-do/.

Stamarski CS, Son Hing LS. Gender inequalities in the workplace: the effects of organizational structures, processes, practices, and decision makers' sexism. Front Psychol. 2015;6:1400. https://doi.org/10.3389/fpsyg.2015.01400.

Vermeulen N, Luyten P. Gender bias in clinical practice: evidence and strategies for change. Int Rev Psychiatry. 2018;30(2):123–32. https://doi.org/10.1080/09540261.2018.1435512.

World Health Organization. Delivered by women, led by men: a gender and equity analysis of the global health and social workforce. WHO; 2019.

LGBTQ+ Inclusivity

5

Introduction to LGBTQ+ Inclusivity in Nursing

Nursing has long been defined by its commitment to compassion, advocacy, and respect for the dignity of every individual (American Nurses Association 2021). These values form the ethical foundation of the profession and are enshrined in its codes of practice worldwide. Yet despite these commitments, healthcare systems including nursing have not always lived up to the promise of inclusivity. One of the clearest examples of this failure lies in the treatment of lesbian, gay, bisexual, transgender, queer, and other sexual and gender minority (LGBTQ+) populations. While the language of equality and respect is frequently invoked, the lived experiences of LGBTQ+ patients and nurses reveal systemic inequities, structural barriers, and interpersonal discrimination that compromise both health outcomes and professional well-being.

LGBTQ+ inclusivity in nursing refers to the intentional creation of care environments, educational systems, and workplace cultures where individuals of all sexual orientations and gender identities are respected, affirmed, and supported (American Nurses Association 2021; Bonvicini 2017). Inclusivity is not merely the absence of overt discrimination but the presence of active practices, policies, and attitudes that ensure equity. For patients, inclusivity means being able to access healthcare without fear of bias, having providers who respect their identities, and receiving care that acknowledges and responds to their unique health needs. For nurses and other healthcare professionals, inclusivity means working in environments where their identities are valued rather than marginalized and where they can contribute fully to the profession without fear of harassment or exclusion.

The importance of inclusivity is underscored by the stark health disparities that LGBTQ+ populations continue to face (Mayer et al. 2008; Institute of Medicine 2011). Compared with heterosexual and cisgender individuals, LGBTQ+ individuals experience higher rates of mental health concerns, substance use, suicide attempts, and certain chronic illnesses. Transgender individuals, in particular,

N. Nami, *Unraveling Social Justice Issues in Nursing*,
https://doi.org/10.1007/978-3-032-26512-8_5

encounter significant barriers to healthcare access, with many reporting instances of being denied care outright, subjected to inappropriate questions, or treated with disrespect. These disparities are not inherent to LGBTQ+ identities but are the direct result of systemic stigma, discrimination, and structural exclusion. Nurses, as frontline providers, are uniquely positioned to mitigate these harms by creating affirming care environments and advocating for systemic reform.

Historically, LGBTQ+ individuals have been marginalized within healthcare systems, often pathologized rather than affirmed (Institute of Medicine 2011; Boehmer 2018). Until 1973, homosexuality was classified as a mental disorder in the Diagnostic and Statistical Manual of Mental Disorders (DSM), a designation that legitimized stigma and medical interventions aimed at "curing" same-sex attraction. Transgender identities were similarly pathologized, with "gender identity disorder" remaining in the DSM until its reclassification as "gender dysphoria" in 2013. These medical frameworks reinforced social discrimination and provided justification for exclusionary practices in healthcare, education, and employment. The legacies of such pathologization persist today, shaping both patient mistrust of healthcare systems and the gaps in providers' education and competence.

For nurses, understanding this history is essential (American Nurses Association 2021; Institute of Medicine 2011). Inclusivity cannot be achieved without acknowledging the ways in which healthcare has historically contributed to the marginalization of LGBTQ+ communities. Moreover, inclusivity requires grappling with the reality that discrimination persists in contemporary practice. Surveys consistently reveal that LGBTQ+ patients anticipate or experience bias in healthcare encounters, leading many to delay or avoid care altogether. Similarly, LGBTQ+ nurses and healthcare staff frequently encounter microaggressions, exclusion from leadership pipelines, and outright discrimination in the workplace. These experiences compromise professional development, morale, and the ability of the workforce to reflect the diversity of the populations it serves.

The ethical foundations of nursing demand a response (American Nurses Association 2021). As mentioned in other chapters, The American Nurses Association's Code of Ethics calls for respect for human dignity, advocacy for vulnerable populations, and a commitment to social justice. These obligations are not abstract; they require concrete action to address the inequities faced by LGBTQ+ patients and professionals. Inclusivity, in this sense, is not optional or peripheral: it is central to nursing's mission. By promoting LGBTQ+ inclusivity, nursing not only fulfills its ethical commitments but also strengthens its ability to provide holistic, person-centered care.

This chapter will explore LGBTQ+ inclusivity in nursing and healthcare across multiple dimensions. It will begin with a discussion of how to create inclusive environments for LGBTQ+ patients, addressing barriers to access and strategies for affirming care (Bonvicini 2017; Bjarnadottir et al. 2017). It will then examine the challenges faced by LGBTQ+ nurses and staff within healthcare institutions, highlighting the need for workplace equity. The chapter will also analyze structural and policy barriers, such as insurance exclusions and inconsistent legal protections, before turning to pathways forward in education, research, advocacy, and institutional accountability. Finally, the conclusion will synthesize these insights and offer a call to action for nursing as a leader in advancing LGBTQ+ equity.

By framing LGBTQ+ inclusivity as both an ethical obligation and a practical necessity, this chapter underscores the urgency of dismantling the barriers that compromise care and professional equity (American Nurses Association 2021; World Health Organization 2013). The health and well-being of LGBTQ+ patients, the dignity of LGBTQ+ nurses, and the credibility of nursing as a profession all depend on the commitment to inclusivity. To ignore these issues is to perpetuate injustice; to confront them is to align nursing with its deepest values of compassion, advocacy, and respect for human dignity.

Creating Inclusive Environments for LGBTQ+ Patients

For LGBTQ+ individuals, the healthcare system has historically been a site of exclusion, stigma, and mistrust (Lambda Legal 2010; Institute of Medicine 2011). Despite progress in civil rights and increased visibility of LGBTQ+ communities, many patients continue to encounter discriminatory practices, structural barriers, and implicit bias that compromise their access to equitable care. Inclusivity in healthcare for LGBTQ+ patients requires more than surface-level tolerance. It demands intentional, systemic, and sustained efforts to create environments where patients feel safe, respected, and empowered to engage fully in their care. Nurses, as frontline providers, are central to this transformation.

One of the most significant barriers LGBTQ+ patients face is fear of discrimination (Whitehead et al. 2016; Lambda Legal 2010). Studies reveal that a substantial proportion of LGBTQ+ individuals avoid seeking healthcare due to concerns about stigma or negative treatment. For example, transgender patients report being denied care outright or subjected to humiliating questions unrelated to their presenting health concerns. Lesbian and bisexual women often receive fewer preventive screenings, such as Pap smears and mammograms, because providers incorrectly assume they are at lower risk. Gay and bisexual men may be disproportionately targeted for HIV-related services while having other health needs overlooked. Such experiences erode trust in healthcare institutions and deter patients from engaging in preventive or ongoing care, perpetuating disparities in health outcomes.

Health disparities among LGBTQ+ populations reflect the cumulative effects of these barriers (National Academies of Sciences, Engineering, and Medicine 2020; Boehmer 2018). Rates of mental health concerns—including depression, anxiety, and suicidality—are higher among LGBTQ+ individuals than among their heterosexual and cisgender peers. LGBTQ+ youth are particularly vulnerable, facing higher risks of bullying, homelessness, and substance use, often linked to rejection by families and communities. Transgender individuals experience disproportionately high rates of attempted suicide, a stark indicator of the impact of stigma, marginalization, and systemic neglect. In addition, LGBTQ+ populations face elevated risks of chronic conditions such as cardiovascular disease, certain cancers, and substance use disorders. These disparities are not the result of intrinsic vulnerabilities but of persistent social and structural inequities that shape health behaviors and access to care.

Creating inclusive environments requires that nurses and healthcare systems actively address these inequities (American Nurses Association 2021; Bonvicini 2017). One foundational step is the use of affirming communication. Respecting patients' chosen names and pronouns is a basic but powerful way of signaling respect and recognition. Failure to do so not only undermines trust but also contributes to the erasure of patients' identities. Nurses must also avoid making assumptions about patients' sexual orientation, gender identity, or family structures. Intake forms and electronic health records should provide inclusive options for documenting identity, allowing patients to self-identify rather than being forced into rigid categories that may not reflect their realities.

Inclusive care also requires the adoption of trauma-informed approaches (Poteat et al. 2013; Bonvicini 2017). Many LGBTQ+ patients have histories of discrimination, rejection, or violence, which can shape how they engage with healthcare providers. Trauma-informed care emphasizes safety, trustworthiness, collaboration, empowerment, and cultural humility. For LGBTQ+ patients, this means creating spaces where disclosure of identity is met with respect, where histories of trauma are acknowledged, and where patients are supported as active participants in their care rather than passive recipients. Nurses are well suited to lead this shift, given their emphasis on holistic and patient-centered care.

Physical environments also play a role in signaling inclusivity (Bonvicini 2017; World Health Organization 2013). Visible symbols of support such as rainbow flags, inclusive posters, or nondiscrimination statements can help LGBTQ+ patients feel safer in clinical settings. More substantively, facilities must ensure privacy in care, provide gender-neutral restrooms, and design spaces that do not reinforce binary assumptions about gender. Training staff at every level of the healthcare system, from receptionists to administrators to clinicians, is essential to ensure that inclusivity is embedded in all interactions, not just those with direct care providers.

In addition to affirming communication and environments, inclusive care requires attention to specific health needs (Mayer et al. 2008; Reisner et al. 2016). For example, while HIV prevention and treatment remain important for men who have sex with men and transgender women, nurses must avoid reducing these populations to single-issue identities. Routine care such as cancer screenings, cardiovascular risk management, and mental health services must be provided without bias or neglect. Similarly, transgender patients may require access to gender-affirming treatments, including hormone therapy and surgical care, but their healthcare needs extend well beyond transition-related services. Nurses must ensure that transgender patients are offered the same preventive and primary care services as other populations, without allowing bias or lack of training to interfere.

Feedback mechanisms are another essential component of inclusive care (Bjarnadottir et al. 2017; National Academies of Sciences, Engineering, and Medicine 2020). Regular input from LGBTQ+ patients and families can help identify gaps in services, highlight areas for improvement, and build accountability into institutions. Patient advisory boards, community partnerships, and targeted surveys can provide valuable insights into how healthcare systems are perceived and experienced. By incorporating LGBTQ+ voices into decision-making processes, institutions move closer to equity and build trust with communities historically excluded from such conversations.

Ultimately, inclusivity for LGBTQ+ patients is not achieved through isolated policies or symbolic gestures but through the consistent practice of respect, equity, and advocacy at every level of care (American Nurses Association 2021; Bonvicini 2017). Nurses must take active responsibility for affirming patients' identities, addressing disparities, and challenging systemic barriers that perpetuate inequity. By doing so, they fulfill their ethical obligations and advance the profession's commitment to justice and holistic care.

Challenges Faced by LGBTQ+ Nurses and Staff

While the discourse on LGBTQ+ inclusivity in healthcare often centers on patients, it is equally important to recognize the realities experienced by LGBTQ+ nurses and healthcare staff (Casey et al. 2019; National Academies of Sciences, Engineering, and Medicine 2020). Nurses not only serve as providers of care but also as members of a workforce that is deeply shaped by the same social forces of stigma, discrimination, and inequity that affect LGBTQ+ communities more broadly. Their professional well-being, opportunities for advancement, and sense of belonging are often compromised by the persistence of homophobia, transphobia, and heteronormative assumptions within healthcare organizations.

One of the most pressing challenges LGBTQ+ nurses face is workplace discrimination (Casey et al. 2019; Lambda Legal 2010). Surveys reveal that LGBTQ+ healthcare workers are more likely than their heterosexual and cisgender peers to report experiences of verbal harassment, exclusion from social networks, and discrimination in promotion or pay. Lesbian and gay nurses may hear derogatory remarks from colleagues or patients, experience pressure to conceal their relationships, or encounter resistance when they advocate for inclusive practices. Transgender and nonbinary nurses frequently report even higher levels of discrimination, ranging from misgendering to outright refusal of colleagues to acknowledge their identities. In environments where inclusivity is lacking, these experiences accumulate into a pervasive climate of exclusion that erodes morale and professional engagement.

Microaggressions also play a significant role in shaping the daily experiences of LGBTQ+ nurses (Baker and Beagan 2014; Casey et al. 2019). These are often subtle or indirect expressions of bias that, while individually dismissible, collectively create a hostile and invalidating environment. Examples include coworkers repeatedly asking invasive questions about a colleague's gender identity or personal relationships, making jokes based on stereotypes, or assuming heterosexuality in casual conversation. Over time, these microaggressions reinforce the message that LGBTQ+ nurses are outsiders in their own workplaces, compelling many to engage in emotional labor to manage or conceal their identities.

Representation in leadership and decision-making remains another barrier (National Academies of Sciences, Engineering, and Medicine 2020; Casey et al. 2019). LGBTQ+ nurses are significantly underrepresented in leadership positions within healthcare organizations and professional associations. The lack of visible role models and mentors contributes to a cycle in which aspiring leaders are discouraged from pursuing advancement, either because they do not see themselves reflected in existing leadership or because they fear increased scrutiny of their identities at higher levels of visibility. This absence of representation not only limits the career trajectories of LGBTQ+ nurses but also perpetuates organizational blind spots regarding inclusivity. Without LGBTQ+ voices at the table, policies, curricula, and organizational strategies may fail to address the specific needs of LGBTQ+ staff and patients.

Balancing professional identity with personal safety presents an ongoing challenge for many LGBTQ+ nurses (Casey et al. 2019; National Academies of Sciences, Engineering, and Medicine 2020). Decisions about whether to disclose one's identity at work are fraught with considerations of risk, support, and vulnerability. While some nurses find affirming workplaces where openness is possible and even celebrated, others face environments where disclosure can lead to ostracization, stalled career progression, or even termination. For transgender nurses, the stakes may be even higher, as transitioning in the workplace can expose individuals to heightened discrimination, harassment, and bureaucratic challenges with benefits or credentialing systems. The psychological toll of navigating these choices between authenticity and safety can contribute to burnout, stress, and decreased job satisfaction.

Intersectionality further complicates the experiences of LGBTQ+ nurses (National Academies of Sciences, Engineering, and Medicine 2020; Casey et al. 2019). For example, a Black lesbian nurse may encounter not only homophobia but also racism and sexism, each compounding the effects of the others. Transgender nurses of color are among the most marginalized, facing systemic barriers in education, employment, and healthcare access while simultaneously navigating discrimination within their workplaces. These intersecting oppressions reveal that the challenges faced by LGBTQ+ nurses cannot be understood in isolation but must be situated within broader systems of inequity.

Despite these challenges, LGBTQ+ nurses have been at the forefront of advocacy and leadership in promoting inclusivity (American Nurses Association 2021; National Academies of Sciences, Engineering, and Medicine 2020). Nursing organizations such as the Gay and Lesbian Medical Association (now GLMA: Health Professionals Advancing LGBTQ+ Equality) and the American Association for Men in Nursing have created networks of support and visibility. Local hospital-based LGBTQ+ employee resource groups provide community and a platform for collective action. However, these initiatives often operate at the margins of larger institutions, and their impact depends heavily on the commitment of organizational leadership. Without structural integration of inclusivity goals into policies and accountability systems, the burden of advocacy often falls disproportionately on LGBTQ+ nurses themselves.

Addressing the challenges faced by LGBTQ+ nurses requires systemic reforms (American Nurses Association 2021; National Academies of Sciences, Engineering, and Medicine 2020). Institutions must adopt comprehensive nondiscrimination policies that explicitly include sexual orientation, gender identity, and gender expression. Anti-bias and inclusivity training must be mandatory, ongoing, and applied at every level of the workforce. Career development programs should intentionally recruit and support LGBTQ+ nurses, creating mentorship pipelines that foster leadership. Perhaps most importantly, organizational cultures must shift toward affirming environments where LGBTQ+ nurses do not merely survive but thrive where authenticity is not punished but valued as a source of strength and diversity.

In conclusion, LGBTQ+ nurses and staff are indispensable members of the healthcare workforce, yet their professional experiences are too often shaped by discrimination, invisibility, and structural inequities (Casey et al. 2019; National Academies of Sciences, Engineering, and Medicine 2020). Ensuring their full inclusion is not only a matter of fairness but also of professional excellence. A nursing workforce that reflects and affirms the diversity of the populations it serves is better equipped to provide compassionate, equitable, and effective care. By dismantling barriers for LGBTQ+ nurses, the profession strengthens both its internal integrity and its external impact, advancing inclusivity as a principle that is lived, not merely stated.

Structural and Policy Barriers

While interpersonal bias and clinical ignorance certainly harm LGBTQ+ patients and staff, the more enduring and far-reaching challenges are rooted in structural and policy barriers (World Health Organization 2013; Reisner et al. 2016). These barriers are embedded in healthcare institutions, insurance systems, and legal frameworks that either fail to protect LGBTQ+ individuals or actively contribute to their marginalization. Understanding these systemic obstacles is essential, because without structural change, even the most well-intentioned individual providers cannot fully eliminate inequities.

One of the most significant structural barriers is insurance exclusion (Reisner et al. 2016; World Health Organization 2013). For decades, many insurance policies explicitly excluded coverage for gender-affirming care such as hormone therapy and gender-affirming surgeries. Even as policies have evolved, coverage remains inconsistent and often subject to arbitrary denials. Patients may face onerous requirements, such as multiple psychiatric evaluations, lengthy waiting periods, or proof of "real-life experience" living in their identified gender before being approved for treatment. These restrictions not only delay care but also reinforce the harmful assumption that transgender and nonbinary identities require external validation before they are legitimate. Beyond gender-affirming care, many LGBTQ+ patients encounter insurance denials for procedures deemed "not medically necessary," such as fertility treatments for same-sex couples, despite their necessity for family building.

Legal protections for LGBTQ+ individuals in healthcare also remain uneven and fragile (World Health Organization 2013; Lambda Legal 2010). In some countries and states, nondiscrimination laws explicitly include sexual orientation, gender identity, and gender expression as protected categories. In others, such protections are absent or contested. Even in jurisdictions where protections exist, enforcement is often weak, leaving individuals vulnerable to discrimination without clear recourse. In the United States, for example, the Affordable Care Act's Section 1557 extended protections against sex discrimination in healthcare, which courts have interpreted to include gender identity and sexual orientation. Yet these protections have been subject to political shifts and legal challenges, creating instability and uncertainty for LGBTQ+ patients and providers. For nurses and other healthcare professionals, this inconsistency complicates the ability to advocate effectively and highlights the need for broader, more durable protections.

Educational institutions and accreditation bodies also contribute to structural inequities by failing to adequately integrate LGBTQ+ health into curricula (Institute of Medicine 2011; National Academies of Sciences, Engineering, and Medicine 2020). Nursing and medical schools often devote limited time to LGBTQ+ topics, leaving graduates underprepared to care for diverse populations. When LGBTQ+ health is addressed, it may be presented as a niche topic rather than a fundamental aspect of person-centered care. This lack of formal education contributes to a cycle in which providers feel unprepared, patients experience inadequate care, and institutions fail to prioritize reform. Accreditation bodies play a key role in setting standards, and their failure to require comprehensive LGBTQ+ education reflects a systemic blind spot that perpetuates inequity across generations of healthcare providers.

Workplace policies similarly reveal structural barriers (Casey et al. 2019; Lambda Legal 2010). Many healthcare institutions lack explicit nondiscrimination policies that protect LGBTQ+ employees, leaving staff vulnerable to harassment and exclusion. Even when policies exist, their enforcement is often inconsistent, with leaders reluctant to challenge powerful stakeholders or entrenched cultural norms. Benefits such as family leave, spousal coverage, and parental rights may not be equitably extended to same-sex partners or LGBTQ+ parents, further institutionalizing disparities. These inequities communicate to LGBTQ+ staff that they are less valued, undermining morale and limiting opportunities for advancement.

Beyond healthcare institutions, broader societal structures also perpetuate inequities that directly impact LGBTQ+ health (World Health Organization 2013; National Academies of Sciences, Engineering, and Medicine 2020). Policies governing housing, employment, and education create social determinants of health that disproportionately disadvantage LGBTQ+ individuals. For instance, discrimination in employment contributes to higher rates of poverty among LGBTQ+ populations, limiting access to healthcare and healthy living conditions. Housing discrimination and rejection by families contribute to high rates of homelessness among LGBTQ+ youth, which in turn exacerbates risks of poor health outcomes. These structural determinants cannot be separated from the role of healthcare providers, as nurses frequently encounter the consequences of these systemic inequities in their clinical practice.

The absence of consistent data collection on sexual orientation and gender identity also represents a structural barrier (Bjarnadottir et al. 2017; National Academies of Sciences, Engineering, and Medicine 2020). Without accurate data, it is difficult to measure disparities, track progress, or develop evidence-based interventions. Many healthcare systems fail to collect this information systematically, either due to lack of training, fear of offending patients, or outdated systems that do not allow for inclusive options. This invisibility in data perpetuates invisibility in policy and practice. Nurses, as leaders in patient assessment and documentation, have a role to play in advocating for respectful and standardized approaches to data collection that affirm patient identities while safeguarding privacy.

Ultimately, structural and policy barriers demonstrate that inequities are not the result of isolated acts of prejudice but are embedded in the very frameworks that govern healthcare delivery and employment (World Health Organization 2013; National Academies of Sciences, Engineering, and Medicine 2020). Addressing these barriers requires systemic reforms at multiple levels: insurance companies must eliminate exclusions and expand equitable coverage; legal protections must be strengthened and consistently enforced; accreditation bodies must mandate LGBTQ+ content in curricula; and healthcare institutions must adopt and enforce robust nondiscrimination and benefits policies. Nurses, as trusted professionals and advocates, have a critical role in pushing for these changes, ensuring that inclusivity is not left to chance or individual goodwill but is embedded in the structures of healthcare itself.

Pathways Toward Equity and Inclusion

If the first step in advancing LGBTQ+ inclusivity is to recognize the barriers that have long shaped health disparities and workplace inequities, the second step is to chart clear and actionable pathways forward (National Academies of Sciences, Engineering, and Medicine 2020; Bonvicini 2017). Inclusivity cannot remain an aspirational goal or a matter of personal goodwill; it must be embedded in the very structures of nursing education, practice, and policy. These pathways toward equity demand a combination of cultural change, institutional reform, and systemic advocacy. Nurses, by virtue of their ethical commitments and trusted positions, are uniquely positioned to lead this effort.

Education is foundational to building inclusivity (Institute of Medicine 2011; Baker and Beagan 2014). For decades, nursing curricula either ignored LGBTQ+ health or relegated it to elective or peripheral content. As a result, generations of nurses graduated without adequate preparation to care for LGBTQ+ patients. To remedy this, LGBTQ+ health must be integrated across the curriculum rather than siloed. This means including content on sexual orientation and gender identity in courses on health assessment, mental health, pediatrics, obstetrics, and geriatrics, as well as embedding cultural humility as a guiding principle throughout nursing education. Simulation exercises, case studies, and community partnerships can help students gain practical competence in affirming care. Furthermore, accreditation bodies must enforce these standards, ensuring that schools of nursing treat LGBTQ+ inclusivity as a core competency rather than an optional add-on.

Research agendas also need to shift to address LGBTQ+ health inequities more systematically (Boehmer 2018; National Academies of Sciences, Engineering, and Medicine 2020). Historically, LGBTQ+ populations have been underrepresented in health research, leading to evidence gaps that perpetuate disparities in care. Nursing research has the potential to fill these gaps by exploring the lived experiences of LGBTQ+ patients, identifying barriers to access, and testing interventions that promote equity. This requires intentional inclusion of LGBTQ+ participants in studies, the development of inclusive methodologies, and funding priorities that recognize the importance of this research. Equally important is ensuring that research findings are translated into practice, informing clinical guidelines, curricula, and policies that affect care delivery.

Policy advocacy remains a crucial pathway to advancing equity (World Health Organization 2013; American Nurses Association 2021). Nurses, individually and collectively, must advocate for nondiscrimination protections at local, national, and international levels. This includes pushing for robust enforcement of existing laws, such as Section 1557 of the Affordable Care Act in the United States, and lobbying for broader protections where gaps remain. Advocacy must also target insurance reforms, ensuring comprehensive coverage for gender-affirming care, fertility treatments, and other services essential to LGBTQ+ patients' health and well-being. At the institutional level, nurses can press for the adoption of explicit nondiscrimination policies, equitable benefits for same-sex partners, and inclusive parental leave policies. These policy shifts create the structural supports necessary to make inclusivity sustainable.

Institutional accountability is another cornerstone of change (National Academies of Sciences, Engineering, and Medicine 2020; Bjarnadottir et al. 2017). Too often, efforts at inclusivity are reduced to symbolic gestures or one-time trainings, without mechanisms for follow-through. Real progress requires that healthcare institutions collect and publish data on LGBTQ+ patients' experiences, track outcomes for LGBTQ+ staff, and create feedback loops that ensure accountability. Patient advisory boards that include LGBTQ+ voices, staff surveys that assess workplace climate, and transparent reporting on inclusivity initiatives can all help to ensure that commitments are more than rhetorical. Nurses, particularly those in leadership, can model accountability by setting measurable goals and reporting progress publicly.

Cultural change within healthcare organizations is equally critical (Baker and Beagan 2014; Bonvicini 2017). Inclusivity requires creating environments where LGBTQ+ patients and staff feel affirmed in their identities, not merely tolerated. This means cultivating a culture of respect, encouraging dialogue about bias, and empowering staff to challenge discriminatory practices when they occur. It also requires dismantling heteronormative and cisnormative assumptions that shape everything from intake forms to hospital visitation policies. Nurses, as the largest and most trusted group of healthcare professionals, play a vital role in shaping this culture. By modeling inclusivity in their everyday practice, mentoring colleagues, and advocating for patients, nurses can help shift organizational norms toward equity.

Finally, building coalitions is essential to sustaining progress (National Academies of Sciences, Engineering, and Medicine 2020; World Health Organization 2013). Inclusivity cannot be advanced by nurses alone; it requires collaboration with patients, community organizations, policymakers, and other healthcare professionals. Community partnerships are particularly powerful, allowing healthcare institutions to learn directly from LGBTQ+ communities about their needs and priorities. Nurses who engage in these partnerships not only build trust but also help bridge the gap between healthcare systems and historically marginalized populations.

Taken together, these pathways, education, research, policy advocacy, accountability, cultural change, and coalition-building, represent a comprehensive strategy for advancing LGBTQ+ inclusivity in nursing and healthcare (National Academies of Sciences, Engineering, and Medicine 2020; American Nurses Association 2021). Each is necessary, and none is sufficient on its own. Progress requires integration across levels, from individual clinical encounters to national policy. For nurses, the call is clear: inclusivity must be lived in daily practice and pursued through systemic change. Only then can nursing fully embody its ethical commitments and ensure that all patients and staff, regardless of sexual orientation or gender identity, experience dignity, respect, and equity.

Conclusion

LGBTQ+ inclusivity in nursing and healthcare is not a matter of political correctness or optional reform; it is central to the profession's ethical obligations and mission (American Nurses Association 2021; Bonvicini 2017). Throughout this chapter, the evidence has shown that LGBTQ+ individuals both patients and professionals continue to experience inequities that compromise health outcomes, workplace safety, and dignity. These inequities are not isolated or incidental but deeply systemic, rooted in histories of pathologization, structural exclusion, and cultural norms that privilege heteronormativity and cisnormativity.

For patients, the consequences of exclusion are stark (Lambda Legal 2010; National Academies of Sciences, Engineering, and Medicine 2020). LGBTQ+ individuals are more likely to delay or avoid care due to fear of discrimination, suffer disproportionate burdens of mental illness and suicide risk, and encounter barriers in accessing basic preventive services as well as gender-affirming care. These disparities are not reflections of LGBTQ+ identities themselves but of the inequities built into healthcare systems that fail to recognize, affirm, and respond to diverse identities. Nurses, who are often the first point of contact and trusted advocates in patient care, hold unique responsibility to counteract these inequities through affirming communication, trauma-informed practice, and advocacy for systemic reform.

For LGBTQ+ nurses and healthcare staff, inequities are just as pervasive (Casey et al. 2019; National Academies of Sciences, Engineering, and Medicine 2020). Experiences of microaggressions, discrimination, and underrepresentation in leadership create hostile work environments that limit opportunities and erode professional well-being. The decision to disclose one's identity in the workplace remains fraught, shaped by fears of exclusion or career repercussions. Without explicit protections, accountability mechanisms, and cultural change, LGBTQ+ nurses are forced to carry the dual burden of caring for others while navigating systemic barriers themselves. Addressing these inequities is essential not only for fairness within the profession but also for strengthening the nursing workforce as a whole.

The analysis of structural and policy barriers demonstrates that inclusivity cannot be left to individual goodwill (World Health Organization 2013; Reisner et al. 2016). Insurance exclusions, inconsistent legal protections, inadequate education, and weak enforcement of nondiscrimination policies perpetuate systemic inequities. Change requires structural reforms, including comprehensive coverage of LGBTQ+ health needs, durable legal protections, accreditation requirements for inclusive curricula, and institutional accountability for equity. Nurses, by engaging in policy advocacy and coalition-building, can ensure that these changes are not peripheral but embedded in the systems that govern healthcare.

The pathways forward such as education, research, policy advocacy, accountability, cultural change, and coalition-building are both ambitious and achievable (National Academies of Sciences, Engineering, and Medicine 2020; Bonvicini 2017). Each requires sustained effort and collaboration, but together they form a comprehensive roadmap toward inclusivity. Nurses, as the largest and most trusted group of healthcare professionals, have both the opportunity and the obligation to lead this transformation. Inclusivity must not remain at the margins of professional practice but must be central to how nursing understands its mission of holistic, person-centered care.

Ultimately, LGBTQ+ inclusivity is about more than addressing disparities (World Health Organization 2013; American Nurses Association 2021). It is about affirming the dignity, worth, and humanity of every individual. It is about ensuring that healthcare is not a site of exclusion but a space of healing and respect. For nursing, it is about living up to its deepest values compassion, advocacy, justice, and respect for human dignity. By committing to LGBTQ+ inclusivity in education, practice, policy, and research, nursing can move beyond rhetoric to reality, transforming both the profession and the lives of those it serves.

References

American Nurses Association. Nursing: scope and standards of practice. 4th ed. American Nurses Association; 2021.

Baker K, Beagan B. Making assumptions, making space: an anthropological critique of cultural competency and its relevance to queer patients. Med Anthropol Q. 2014;28(4):578–98. https://doi.org/10.1111/maq.12129.

Bjarnadottir RI, Bockting W, Dowding DW. Patient perspectives on answering questions about sexual orientation and gender identity: an integrative review. J Clin Nurs. 2017;26(13–14):1814–33. https://doi.org/10.1111/jocn.13612.

Boehmer U. Twenty years of public health research: inclusion of lesbian, gay, bisexual, and transgender populations. Am J Publ Health. 2018;102(7):1349–56. https://doi.org/10.2105/AJPH.2011.300388.

Bonvicini KA. LGBT healthcare disparities: what progress have we made? Patient Educ Couns. 2017;100(12):2357–61. https://doi.org/10.1016/j.pec.2017.06.003.

Casey LS, Reisner SL, Findling MG, Blendon RJ, Benson JM, Sayde JM, Miller C. Discrimination in the United States: experiences of lesbian, gay, bisexual, transgender, and queer Americans. Health Serv Res. 2019;54(S2):1454–66. https://doi.org/10.1111/1475-6773.13229.

Institute of Medicine. The health of lesbian, gay, bisexual, and transgender people: building a foundation for better understanding. National Academies Press; 2011. https://doi.org/10.17226/13128.

Lambda Legal. When health care isn't caring: Lambda Legal's survey of discrimination against LGBT people and people with HIV. Lambda Legal; 2010.

Mayer KH, Bradford JB, Makadon HJ, Stall R, Goldhammer H, Landers S. Sexual and gender minority health: what we know and what needs to be done. Am J Publ Health. 2008;98(6):989–95. https://doi.org/10.2105/AJPH.2007.127811.

National Academies of Sciences, Engineering, and Medicine. Understanding the well-being of LGBTQI+ populations. National Academies Press. 2020; https://doi.org/10.17226/25877.

Poteat T, German D, Kerrigan D. Managing uncertainty: a grounded theory of stigma in transgender health care encounters. Soc Sci Med. 2013;84:22–9. https://doi.org/10.1016/j.socscimed.2013.02.019.

Reisner SL, Radix A, Deutsch MB. Integrated and gender-affirming transgender clinical care and research. J Acquir Immune Defic Syndr. 2016;72(S3):S235–42. https://doi.org/10.1097/QAI.0000000000001088.

Whitehead J, Shaver J, Stephenson R. Outness, stigma, and primary health care utilization among rural LGBT populations. PLoS One. 2016;11(1):e0146139. https://doi.org/10.1371/journal.pone.0146139.

World Health Organization. Addressing the causes of disparities in health service access and utilization for lesbian, gay, bisexual and trans (LGBT) persons. WHO; 2013.

Socioeconomic Inequalities 6

Introduction to Socioeconomic Inequalities in Healthcare

Socioeconomic inequality has long been recognized as one of the most powerful determinants of health (Marmot 2005; Braveman and Gottlieb 2014). While healthcare often focuses on individual pathology and biological risk factors, a growing body of research shows that the conditions in which people are born, grow, live, work, and age shape their health outcomes more profoundly than any single clinical intervention. These social determinants of health particularly income, education, employment, housing, and neighborhood conditions create an uneven playing field that places individuals from lower socioeconomic backgrounds at a systematic disadvantage. For nurses, whose professional mandate emphasizes holistic and equitable care, understanding and addressing these inequalities is not simply an academic exercise but a moral and ethical imperative.

Socioeconomic status (SES) is generally defined by three interrelated components: income, education, and occupation (Cockerham 2021; Graham 2007). Each of these dimensions influences health in direct and indirect ways. Low-income limits access to nutritious food, safe housing, and quality healthcare. Limited education constrains employment opportunities and health literacy, making it more difficult for individuals to navigate complex health systems. Occupational status shapes both income and exposure to health risks, with low-wage jobs often associated with unsafe working conditions, limited benefits, and high levels of stress. Together, these factors create a cumulative disadvantage that compounds over the life course, contributing to stark differences in morbidity and mortality across socioeconomic groups.

The historical roots of socioeconomic inequalities in healthcare are deeply entwined with broader systems of social stratification (Farmer 2004; Raphael 2016). In the United States, for example, access to healthcare has long been tied to employment and private insurance, a structure that inherently disadvantages those in precarious or low-wage work. Similar patterns can be seen globally, where neoliberal

N. Nami, *Unraveling Social Justice Issues in Nursing*,
https://doi.org/10.1007/978-3-032-26512-8_6

economic policies, austerity measures, and underfunded public health systems have left marginalized communities with inadequate healthcare access. These historical and structural dynamics remind us that socioeconomic inequalities are not natural or inevitable but the result of political and policy choices.

The consequences of socioeconomic inequality are evident across a wide spectrum of health outcomes (Marmot 2005; Braveman et al. 2011). Individuals living in poverty have higher rates of chronic conditions such as diabetes, hypertension, and cardiovascular disease. They experience greater mental health burdens, with poverty closely linked to depression, anxiety, and substance use disorders. Maternal and child health outcomes are particularly sensitive to socioeconomic disparities, with higher rates of low birthweight, infant mortality, and maternal complications among low-income populations. These disparities persist across generations, creating cycles of disadvantage that are difficult to break without systemic intervention.

For nursing, the significance of socioeconomic inequality is twofold (American Nurses Association 2015; Braveman and Gottlieb 2014). First, nurses care for patients across the socioeconomic spectrum, often serving as the first point of contact for individuals who face significant barriers to healthcare access. Nurses witness firsthand the effects of poverty on health, whether it is a patient who cannot afford prescribed medication, a family struggling with food insecurity, or a community with limited access to preventive care. Second, nurses themselves are embedded in healthcare systems shaped by socioeconomic inequalities. They encounter structural barriers such as underfunded hospitals, staffing shortages, and limited community resources that constrain their ability to deliver equitable care. These realities underscore the interconnectedness of patient well-being, nursing practice, and broader socioeconomic conditions.

The ethical foundations of nursing emphasize justice, advocacy, and respect for human dignity (American Nurses Association 2015). The American Nurses Association (ANA) Code of Ethics explicitly calls on nurses to advocate for social justice in health policy and to work toward the elimination of health disparities. Addressing socioeconomic inequality aligns directly with this mandate. To ignore the role of SES in shaping health outcomes is to neglect one of the most fundamental drivers of inequity. Nurses must therefore expand their scope of practice beyond the bedside to include advocacy for systemic change, engaging with policy, community organizations, and interdisciplinary partners to confront the root causes of health disparities.

Globally, the World Health Organization (WHO) has highlighted the importance of reducing health inequities as a moral imperative and a matter of social justice (World Health Organization 2008; Marmot et al. 2008). In its landmark report, Closing the Gap in a Generation, the WHO Commission on Social Determinants of Health emphasized that inequities are not the result of biological fate but of "the inequitable distribution of power, money, and resources.". This framing is crucial because it shifts responsibility away from individuals and places it squarely on the systems and structures that shape health opportunities. For nursing, adopting this perspective challenges practitioners to see beyond individual patient behaviors and to address the broader contexts that influence health.

In this chapter, socioeconomic inequalities in healthcare will be explored in depth, beginning with an examination of how SES shapes health outcomes, moving through barriers to care, and analyzing the specific challenges faced by nurses in addressing these disparities. Strategies for bridging the socioeconomic gap will be considered, drawing on evidence from policy, nursing practice, and community-based interventions (Braveman et al. 2011; World Health Organization 2008). The chapter will conclude by framing socioeconomic justice as inseparable from nursing ethics, arguing that to fulfill the profession's mission, nurses must commit to dismantling the systemic inequalities that undermine health equity.

How SES Shapes Health Outcomes

The relationship between socioeconomic status and health outcomes is one of the most consistent findings in public health research (Marmot 2005; Braveman et al. 2011). Across countries, populations, and time periods, individuals with lower SES experience higher rates of illness, disability, and premature death than their more affluent counterparts. These patterns persist even in nations with universal health systems, suggesting that the impact of SES extends far beyond access to medical care alone. It reflects a complex interplay of material deprivation, psychosocial stress, and cumulative disadvantage that shapes health over the life course.

Income inequality is perhaps the most visible dimension of SES affecting health (Robert Wood Johnson Foundation 2016; Braveman and Gottlieb 2014). Individuals with low income face direct barriers to accessing healthcare services, from difficulty affording medications to inability to pay for preventive screenings. Yet income also affects health in subtler ways. Poorer households often live in neighborhoods with higher exposure to environmental hazards, such as air pollution, lead, or unsafe drinking water. They are more likely to experience food insecurity, limiting access to nutritious diets necessary for disease prevention. Housing instability and unsafe living conditions further contribute to poor physical and mental health. These material deprivations are not isolated risks but interlocking disadvantages that amplify one another.

Education plays a central role in shaping health outcomes through both knowledge and opportunity (Braveman et al. 2011; Cockerham 2021). Educational attainment is strongly associated with health literacy, which influences the ability to understand health information, navigate healthcare systems, and adhere to treatment regimens. Individuals with limited education may be less able to interpret prescription labels, less comfortable questioning providers, and less aware of preventive services available to them. Beyond health literacy, education opens pathways to stable employment and higher income, which in turn provide resources for healthy living. Conversely, limited education narrows opportunities and entrenches disadvantage, perpetuating cycles of poor health across generations.

Occupation represents another pathway linking SES to health (Cockerham 2021; Marmot 2005). Jobs vary widely in their physical demands, safety standards, benefits, and levels of stress. Low-wage workers often hold jobs in industries with high risks of injury, toxic exposure, or repetitive strain, yet they may lack access to health insurance, sick leave, or disability protections. The stress of job insecurity, workplace discrimination, or exploitation contributes to chronic stress, which has been linked to cardiovascular disease, weakened immune function, and mental health problems. By contrast, higher-status occupations often confer not only better pay and benefits but also a sense of autonomy and control, factors strongly correlated with better health outcomes.

The cumulative effects of SES disparities over the life course produce what scholars term a "health gradient," whereby each step down the socioeconomic ladder is associated with worse health outcomes (Marmot 2005; Graham 2007). This gradient begins in childhood, as children born into poverty are more likely to experience malnutrition, inadequate healthcare, and exposure to toxic stress, all of which affect physical and cognitive development. These disadvantages set the stage for lower educational attainment, poorer employment prospects, and increased health risks in adulthood. By middle age, the cumulative toll of these factors manifests in higher rates of chronic disease, and by later life, in reduced life expectancy. Importantly, the health gradient is not only about poverty versus wealth, it affects every rung of the ladder, meaning that even moderate disadvantages can result in measurable differences in health.

Mental health is also deeply intertwined with SES (Graham 2007; Raphael 2016). The stress of financial insecurity, unemployment, and social marginalization is strongly correlated with depression, anxiety, and substance use disorders. Poverty can exacerbate the effects of trauma, limit access to mental health services, and contribute to stigma that prevents individuals from seeking help. Conversely, untreated mental illness can undermine educational attainment, employability, and financial stability, creating a vicious cycle of disadvantage. Nurses working in mental health settings often encounter the compounded effects of SES and stigma, making socioeconomic sensitivity essential to effective care.

The role of SES in shaping maternal and child health outcomes is particularly striking (World Health Organization 2008; Marmot et al. 2008). Research consistently shows that women with lower SES are more likely to experience complications during pregnancy, receive inadequate prenatal care, and give birth to infants with low birthweight. These disparities are not solely the result of individual behaviors but are linked to structural inequalities, such as lack of access to nutritious food, unsafe housing, and limited healthcare services. For children, early exposure to poverty is associated with higher rates of developmental delays, chronic illness, and academic difficulties, perpetuating intergenerational cycles of disadvantage. Nurses in obstetric, pediatric, and community health settings therefore play a crucial role in identifying and mitigating these risks.

Intergenerational effects of SES further underscore the depth of its impact (Raphael 2016; Cockerham 2021). Health disparities are not only experienced by individuals in the present but also transmitted across generations. Children raised in poverty are more likely to experience poor health as adults, and adults in poor health are more likely to experience downward mobility, further disadvantaging their children. This cycle demonstrates that socioeconomic inequality is not merely a snapshot of the present but a dynamic process that shapes future generations' health prospects. Breaking this cycle requires interventions that address both immediate needs and structural causes of inequality.

The mechanisms through which SES shapes health are complex and multifaceted, involving biological, behavioral, environmental, and social pathways (Cockerham 2021; Marmot 2005). Chronic stress associated with poverty, for example, has measurable biological effects on the hypothalamic-pituitary-adrenal (HPA) axis, leading to dysregulation of cortisol and increased vulnerability to disease. Limited financial resources may constrain health-related behaviors, such as diet and exercise, while unsafe neighborhoods may make outdoor activity impractical or unsafe. At the societal level, structural inequities in funding for schools, healthcare systems, and housing reinforce these disadvantages, making it difficult for individuals to escape their circumstances.

For nurses, recognizing the profound influence of SES on health outcomes requires a shift in perspective (American Nurses Association 2015; Braveman and Gottlieb 2014). Rather than framing patients' health solely in terms of individual choices, nurses must adopt a broader lens that accounts for the structural and social factors shaping those choices. This perspective does not absolve individuals of agency but acknowledges that agency is constrained by context. A patient with diabetes who struggles to manage their diet, for instance, may not lack willpower but rather access to affordable healthy food. A patient who misses appointments may be limited not by motivation but by unreliable transportation. By identifying these structural barriers, nurses can provide more compassionate, realistic, and effective care.

In conclusion, socioeconomic status exerts a powerful influence on health outcomes through interconnected pathways of income, education, and occupation, compounded over the life course and across generations (Marmot 2005; Cockerham 2021). The disparities that result are not natural or inevitable but reflect broader social inequalities that must be addressed at both the clinical and policy levels. For nursing, this means not only treating illness but also advocating for the systemic changes needed to create a more equitable distribution of health opportunities.

Barriers to Healthcare Access for Low-SES Populations

Access to healthcare is often framed in terms of availability whether services exist in a given community, but for low-socioeconomic-status (SES) populations, the barriers are far more complex (Braveman and Gottlieb 2014; World Health Organization 2008). Access is not simply about whether clinics or hospitals exist; it is about whether individuals can afford care, whether they can physically reach it, whether they feel welcomed and respected when they arrive, and whether systemic structures support continuity of care over time. For low-income families, these barriers compound one another, creating a landscape in which obtaining even basic preventive or urgent healthcare can become an overwhelming challenge.

Financial barriers remain the most immediate and visible obstacle (Robert Wood Johnson Foundation 2016; Braveman et al. 2011). Even in countries with public healthcare systems, costs associated with transportation, medications, and time off work can prevent people from seeking care. In the United States, where insurance coverage is tied largely to employment, low-wage workers often fall into coverage gaps. They may earn too much to qualify for Medicaid but too little to afford private insurance premiums, creating a situation of underinsurance that leaves families vulnerable to catastrophic medical debt. Even those with insurance may avoid seeking care due to high deductibles, copayments, or uncovered services. These financial pressures mean that low-SES patients frequently delay seeking care until conditions worsen, contributing to higher rates of emergency department use and preventable hospitalizations.

Transportation and geographic barriers further complicate access (Solar and Irwin 2010; World Health Organization 2008). Many rural areas, where poverty rates are disproportionately high, lack adequate healthcare infrastructure, forcing residents to travel long distances for basic services. Public transportation options are often limited or nonexistent, particularly for those in suburban or rural communities. For urban residents, inadequate or unsafe transit systems can pose similar challenges. Without reliable transportation, routine appointments, follow-ups, and preventive screenings are often missed, undermining health outcomes. Nurses working in community health frequently identify transportation as one of the most significant obstacles patients face, particularly for elderly patients, those with disabilities, or families juggling multiple jobs.

Food insecurity represents another critical barrier linked to socioeconomic inequality (Robert Wood Johnson Foundation 2016; Raphael 2016). Healthy nutrition is foundational to disease prevention and management, yet access to affordable, nutritious food is far from guaranteed for low-income households. Many communities are classified as "food deserts," lacking grocery stores that sell fresh produce or healthy options. Instead, residents may rely on fast food outlets or convenience stores with limited, high-calorie, low-nutrient options. For patients with chronic conditions such as diabetes or hypertension, these food environments make it nearly impossible to adhere to dietary recommendations. Nurses often encounter patients whose ability to manage their health is constrained not by lack of knowledge but by structural barriers to accessing healthy food.

The digital divide increasingly contributes to healthcare disparities as well (Solar and Irwin 2010; Robert Wood Johnson Foundation 2016). With the expansion of telehealth, digital literacy and access to technology have become prerequisites for participation in healthcare. Yet low-income families may lack broadband Internet, smartphones, or the technical skills to navigate online platforms. This exclusion is particularly harmful for populations in rural areas or for those requiring frequent follow-up care. Nurses and providers may assume that patients can receive reminders via email or participate in telehealth appointments, but for many low-SES patients, these assumptions reflect privilege rather than reality. Without deliberate efforts to address the digital divide, telehealth risks reinforcing rather than reducing disparities.

Cultural and systemic barriers compound these structural inequities (Farmer 2004; Braveman and Gottlieb 2014). Low-SES patients often report feeling stigmatized or disrespected in healthcare encounters, with providers attributing health problems to personal failings rather than structural disadvantage. Such attitudes can discourage patients from seeking care, reinforcing cycles of avoidance and mistrust. Language barriers and limited health literacy further undermine patients' ability to engage effectively with healthcare systems. For immigrant populations, fears about documentation status or discrimination may deter families from seeking care altogether. Nurses who practice cultural humility and advocacy play a vital role in counteracting these barriers, yet they often work within systems that perpetuate them.

Case studies of urban versus rural disparities further illustrate these challenges (World Health Organization 2008; Solar and Irwin 2010). In urban centers, healthcare facilities may be more numerous, but overcrowding, underfunding, and staff shortages create long wait times and limited continuity of care. Low-income patients may rely on safety-net hospitals or federally qualified health centers, which provide essential services but often lack resources to meet overwhelming demand. In rural areas, the absence of healthcare facilities altogether may force patients to drive hours for emergency services or prenatal care, with devastating consequences for outcomes such as maternal mortality. These geographic inequities intersect with race, class, and immigration status, producing a layered landscape of disadvantage.

Taken together, these barriers financial, geographic, nutritional, digital, cultural, and systemic reveal that access to healthcare for low-SES populations is not a single issue but a constellation of interrelated challenges (Braveman and Gottlieb 2014; Solar and Irwin 2010). For nurses, addressing these barriers requires more than clinical expertise; it demands advocacy, creativity, and systemic thinking. Whether by arranging transportation assistance, connecting patients to food banks, providing information in plain language, or lobbying for expanded Medicaid coverage, nurses are on the frontlines of mitigating the effects of socioeconomic inequality on healthcare access. Yet until systemic reforms address the root causes, these efforts remain stopgap measures in the face of pervasive inequities.

Socioeconomic Inequalities in Nursing Practice

While socioeconomic inequalities manifest most visibly in the lives of patients, they also deeply shape the practice of nursing (American Nurses Association 2015; Farmer 2004). Nurses are often caught in the middle responsible for delivering equitable and compassionate care while working within healthcare systems constrained by funding shortages, structural inequities, and political decisions beyond their control. This tension highlights the dual role of nurses: they are both witnesses to the consequences of socioeconomic inequality and actors whose capacity to respond is shaped by the very same systemic forces.

One of the most pressing ways socioeconomic inequalities affect nursing practice is through resource limitations (Farmer 2004; World Health Organization 2008).

Underfunded hospitals and clinics, particularly those serving low-income or rural communities, often operate with inadequate staffing, outdated equipment, and insufficient supplies. Nurses in these settings face overwhelming patient loads, long shifts, and high stress, conditions that increase the risk of burnout and turnover. When staffing levels are inadequate, nurses are forced to triage care, prioritizing urgent needs while deferring preventive or holistic interventions. This compromises the quality of care delivered and leaves both patients and providers dissatisfied. The systemic under-resourcing of healthcare institutions that serve disadvantaged populations is a direct reflection of broader socioeconomic inequalities, as wealthier areas typically attract greater investment and political support.

Nurses also encounter socioeconomic barriers in the form of patients' unmet social needs (Braveman and Gottlieb 2014; Robert Wood Johnson Foundation 2016). Daily practice often involves far more than clinical tasks; it requires helping patients navigate complex webs of poverty, housing insecurity, food scarcity, and transportation barriers. For example, a nurse discharging a patient with heart failure may know that dietary changes and regular follow-ups are essential, but if the patient lacks access to healthy food or reliable transportation, the nurse must decide how much time and energy to devote to finding community resources, arranging social work referrals, or advocating for system-level supports. These challenges stretch the scope of nursing and highlight the profession's frontline role in addressing social determinants of health.

Ethically, the profession calls on nurses to advocate for justice and equity (American Nurses Association 2015). The American Nurses Association (ANA) Code of Ethics states that nurses must promote social justice in health policy and advocate for the elimination of health disparities. Yet the gap between this ethical ideal and the daily realities of practice can be immense. Nurses working in resource-poor settings often feel torn between their commitment to patients and the systemic barriers that prevent them from meeting those patients' needs. This ethical tension can lead to moral distress, in which nurses feel powerless to provide the care they know is necessary. Over time, moral distress erodes professional satisfaction and contributes to attrition in already under-resourced communities, perpetuating cycles of inequity.

Nursing education, too, reflects and reinforces socioeconomic inequalities (Cockerham 2021; Raphael 2016). Students from low-income backgrounds often face barriers to entering or completing nursing programs, from the high cost of tuition and textbooks to the need to balance work and caregiving responsibilities. Those who graduate may carry significant student debt, limiting their career choices and pushing them toward higher-paying specialties rather than community or primary care. This creates workforce imbalances that exacerbate existing inequities, as underserved communities struggle to recruit and retain nurses. Furthermore, nursing programs may fail to adequately prepare students to recognize and address the socioeconomic determinants of health, leaving new graduates ill-equipped to respond to the challenges they will inevitably encounter in practice.

The working conditions of nurses also mirror broader socioeconomic divides (Farmer 2004; Cockerham 2021). Nurses in affluent hospitals may have access to advanced technology, robust staffing, and institutional support, while those in safety-net hospitals often face crumbling infrastructure and minimal resources. These disparities are not only unfair to staff but also directly impact patient outcomes, as research consistently shows that nurse staffing levels and working conditions are correlated with quality of care. In this way, socioeconomic inequality in nursing practice is a matter of both workforce justice and patient safety.

Importantly, nurses themselves are not immune to socioeconomic vulnerabilities (Cockerham 2021; Graham 2007). While the profession is often seen as stable and well-paying, many nurses particularly licensed practical nurses (LPNs), home health aides, and nursing assistants earn modest wages and face significant job insecurity. These workers are disproportionately women and people of color, and they often work multiple jobs to support their families. For these nurses, socioeconomic inequality is not an abstract concept but a lived reality. They experience firsthand the stress of inadequate pay, limited benefits, and unsafe working conditions, even as they provide care to patients facing similar struggles. This dual burden highlights the need for nursing advocacy not only for patients but also for the profession itself.

Socioeconomic inequality also shapes how nurses engage in advocacy (American Nurses Association 2015; World Health Organization 2008). Those working in well-resourced institutions may have the time, support, and platforms to participate in policy discussions, professional organizations, or research initiatives. In contrast, nurses in underfunded settings may be too overwhelmed by day-to-day demands to engage in broader systemic change. This uneven distribution of advocacy capacity perpetuates inequities, as the voices of those most affected by socioeconomic disparities are often the least represented in decision-making arenas.

In summary, socioeconomic inequalities permeate nursing practice at every level: the resources available to institutions, the daily realities of patient care, the ethical dilemmas nurses face, the accessibility of nursing education, and the working conditions of the profession itself (American Nurses Association 2015; Cockerham 2021). Nurses are both witnesses to and participants in these inequities, positioned at the intersection of individual suffering and systemic injustice. Addressing these inequalities requires not only individual resilience but systemic transformation greater investment in safety-net institutions, equitable access to nursing education, improved working conditions, and stronger advocacy structures. Only then can nurses fulfill their ethical mandate to promote justice and equity in healthcare.

Strategies for Bridging the Socioeconomic Gap

Confronting socioeconomic inequalities in healthcare requires more than recognition of their existence; it demands intentional strategies to reduce disparities and create systems that are both accessible and equitable (Marmot et al. 2008; Braveman and Gottlieb 2014). While the roots of inequality are structural and far-reaching, solutions can emerge at multiple levels policy reform, institutional accountability, community partnership, and individual nursing practice. Nurses play a critical role in this effort, not only by providing direct patient care but by leveraging their professional authority to advocate for systemic change.

Policy solutions remain among the most powerful tools for reducing health disparities (World Health Organization 2008; Marmot et al. 2008). Expansions of public insurance programs, such as Medicaid in the United States, have been shown to improve access to care for low-income populations, reduce rates of uninsurance, and narrow racial and socioeconomic health disparities. Universal coverage systems, where implemented, have demonstrated significant improvements in equity, ensuring that healthcare is not contingent on employment or income. Yet policy solutions must go beyond insurance alone. Investments in public health infrastructure, housing, education, and social safety nets address the upstream determinants of health that shape outcomes long before patients enter a clinic. Nurses, as trusted professionals and the largest sector of the healthcare workforce, can amplify calls for such reforms, testifying to the consequences of policy decisions at the bedside and in the community.

At the level of healthcare institutions, strategies must prioritize equity in both access and quality of care (Braveman et al. 2011; American Nurses Association 2015). Hospitals and clinics serving disadvantaged populations require greater financial investment, not less, to ensure they can meet the needs of their communities. Equitable funding formulas, culturally responsive care models, and workforce incentives to recruit and retain nurses in underserved areas are crucial. Safety-net hospitals, federally qualified health centers, and community clinics must be recognized not as charity services but as essential infrastructure deserving of sustained support. Nurses within these institutions can advocate for equitable resource allocation, identify gaps in service delivery, and collaborate with administrators to design programs that meet patients where they are.

Nursing practice itself offers numerous avenues for addressing socioeconomic disparities (American Nurses Association 2015; Braveman and Gottlieb 2014). One increasingly important approach is the systematic screening of patients for social determinants of health. Tools integrated into electronic health records can prompt nurses to ask about food insecurity, housing instability, transportation barriers, or financial stress. When identified, these needs can be linked to community resources, such as food pantries, rental assistance programs, or ride services. While these interventions do not eliminate the underlying causes of inequality, they help mitigate its effects and ensure that patients' health plans are realistic and achievable. Such approaches reframe nursing care as not merely clinical but also social, affirming the holistic nature of the profession.

Care coordination and case management are additional strategies nurses can use to support patients facing socioeconomic barriers (American Nurses Association 2015; Braveman et al. 2011). By coordinating between primary care providers, specialists, social workers, and community organizations, nurses can help patients navigate complex health systems that might otherwise overwhelm them. For patients with chronic conditions, this support can be life-changing, reducing hospital readmissions, improving medication adherence, and enhancing quality of life. Importantly, these strategies require institutional support in the form of adequate staffing, training, and recognition of the value of such roles.

Community partnerships represent another essential strategy for bridging socioeconomic gaps (Raphael 2016; Solar and Irwin 2010). Health does not occur in isolation; it is shaped by the environments in which people live. Collaborating with schools, housing authorities, faith-based organizations, and local nonprofits allows nurses and healthcare institutions to extend their reach beyond the clinic walls. Community health worker programs, for example, employ individuals from the community to provide culturally relevant support and education, bridging trust gaps between patients and providers. Nurses can play a leadership role in designing, supervising, and collaborating with such programs, ensuring that interventions are grounded in the lived realities of the populations they serve.

Education and training within nursing must also evolve to prepare professionals for the complexities of socioeconomic disparities (American Nurses Association 2015; Braveman and Gottlieb 2014). Nursing curricula should incorporate robust content on health equity, social determinants of health, and policy advocacy. Clinical rotations in underserved communities can provide students with firsthand exposure to the challenges of poverty and structural inequality, fostering empathy and equipping future nurses with the skills to address such challenges. Continuing education for practicing nurses can further reinforce these competencies, ensuring that equity remains a professional priority throughout one's career.

Finally, interdisciplinary collaboration is indispensable (Solar and Irwin 2010; World Health Organization 2008). Physicians, social workers, public health professionals, educators, and policymakers all play roles in addressing socioeconomic inequality. Nurses, with their holistic perspective and close patient relationships, are ideally positioned to serve as connectors across disciplines. By participating in interdisciplinary teams, nurses can advocate for patients' needs while ensuring that care plans account for social as well as medical factors. Collaborative approaches are particularly effective in addressing complex issues such as homelessness, substance use, and chronic disease management, where no single profession can provide a complete solution.

Taken together, these strategies policy reforms, institutional investment, nursing interventions, community partnerships, educational innovations, and interdisciplinary collaboration form a multifaceted response to socioeconomic inequality in healthcare (Marmot et al. 2008; Braveman and Gottlieb 2014). None of these solutions is sufficient on its own, but when combined, they create pathways toward equity that honor the dignity and worth of all patients. Nurses, by embracing their roles as clinicians, advocates, educators, and leaders, are essential to realizing this vision.

Conclusion

Socioeconomic inequality is one of the most pervasive and persistent forces shaping health outcomes (Marmot 2005; World Health Organization 2008). From the cradle to the grave, socioeconomic status determines who thrives and who struggles, who has access to care and who is left behind, who enjoys long life expectancy and who faces premature death. These inequities are not incidental or unavoidable; they are produced and reproduced by structures that distribute resources, opportunities, and risks unequally across society. For nursing, a profession grounded in justice, compassion, and advocacy, ignoring these inequalities, would mean failing to live up to its ethical obligations.

Throughout this chapter, the pathways through which socioeconomic status shapes health outcomes have been made clear (Braveman et al. 2011; Cockerham 2021). Income, education, and occupation converge to create cumulative disadvantage that manifests in chronic disease, poor maternal and child health, mental health struggles, and reduced life expectancy. The barriers faced by low-SES populations financial hardship, transportation challenges, food insecurity, digital exclusion, and cultural stigmatization are not matters of individual failure but of systemic neglect. Nurses encounter these realities daily, both in their patients' lives and in the conditions of their own practice, which are too often constrained by resource scarcity and institutional inequities.

Yet, the narrative of socioeconomic inequality in healthcare is not solely one of despair (Braveman and Gottlieb 2014; World Health Organization 2008). There are proven strategies for bridging these gaps: expanding insurance coverage, strengthening public health infrastructure, screening for social determinants of health, coordinating care across sectors, and building partnerships with communities. Nursing education is evolving to prepare professionals to engage with these complexities, while research increasingly documents the ways inequities operate and how they might be dismantled. The profession itself has demonstrated resilience and leadership, with nurses using their trusted voices to call for reforms that align healthcare with equity and justice.

What emerges most strongly is the recognition that addressing socioeconomic inequality is not an optional or peripheral aspect of nursing: it is central to its mission (American Nurses Association 2015; Braveman and Gottlieb 2014). Advocacy for health equity is not separate from providing care; it is part of providing care. Every encounter with a patient struggling to afford medication, every referral for housing assistance, every act of policy advocacy on behalf of marginalized communities embodies nursing's commitment to justice. Nurses cannot treat illness effectively without also confronting the conditions that produce it.

The task ahead is formidable (World Health Organization 2008; Raphael 2016). Socioeconomic inequality is deeply entrenched, shaped by centuries of policy, culture, and economics. Change will not come quickly or easily. But nursing is uniquely positioned to contribute to this change because it bridges the worlds of policy and practice, science and compassion, clinical care and social justice. By committing to dismantling socioeconomic barriers, nurses reaffirm their role as advocates for human dignity and stewards of equity.

Ultimately, confronting socioeconomic inequality requires a reimagining of healthcare itself (Solar and Irwin 2010; Marmot et al. 2008; Williams et al. 2019). Systems must move beyond treating disease toward creating conditions in which all people can live healthy, dignified lives. Nursing, with its holistic vision and unwavering commitment to the vulnerable, can lead this transformation. The profession's challenge and its greatest opportunity is to ensure that health is not a privilege of wealth but a right enjoyed by all.

References

American Nurses Association. Code of ethics for nurses with interpretive statements. American Nurses Association; 2015.

Braveman P, Gottlieb L. The social determinants of health: it's time to consider the causes of the causes. Public Health Rep. 2014;129(1_suppl2):19–31. https://doi.org/10.1177/00333549141291S206.

Braveman P, Egerter S, Williams DR. The social determinants of health: coming of age. Annu Rev Public Health. 2011;32(1):381–98. https://doi.org/10.1146/annurev-publhealth-031210-101218.

Cockerham WC. Social causes of health and disease. 3rd ed. Polity Press; 2021.

Farmer P. An anthropology of structural violence. Curr Anthropol. 2004;45(3):305–25. https://doi.org/10.1086/382250.

Graham H. Unequal lives: health and socioeconomic inequalities. Open University Press; 2007.

Marmot M. Social determinants of health inequalities. Lancet. 2005;365:1099–104. https://doi.org/10.1016/S0140-6736(05)74234-3.

Marmot M, Friel S, Bell R, Houweling TA, Taylor S. Closing the gap in a generation: health equity through action on the social determinants of health. Lancet. 2008;372(9650):1661–9. https://doi.org/10.1016/S0140-6736(08)61690-6.

Raphael D. Social determinants of health: Canadian perspectives. 3rd ed. Canadian Scholars' Press; 2016.

Robert Wood Johnson Foundation. Income, wealth and health: exploring the socioeconomic pathways to health equity. Robert Wood Johnson Foundation; 2016.

Solar O, Irwin A. A conceptual framework for action on the social determinants of health. World Health Organization; 2010.

Williams DR, Lawrence JA, Davis BA. Racism and health: evidence and needed research. Annu Rev Public Health. 2019;40:105–25. https://doi.org/10.1146/annurev-publhealth-040218-043750.

World Health Organization. Closing the gap in a generation: health equity through action on the social determinants of health. WHO Commission on Social Determinants of Health; 2008.

Mental Health Stigma

7

Introduction to Mental Health Stigma

Stigma surrounding mental illness has long been one of the most intractable barriers to achieving equitable healthcare (Corrigan and Watson 2002; Henderson et al. 2013). Unlike many physical health conditions, mental illness carries with it not only the burden of symptoms but also the weight of negative stereotypes, social exclusion, and systemic discrimination. Stigma manifests both overtly, through acts of prejudice and exclusion, and subtly, through microaggressions, silence, or dismissive attitudes. For patients, this means that seeking help often comes at the cost of social judgment, loss of status, or fear of being labeled. For nurses and other healthcare professionals, it creates moral and ethical challenges, shaping both how care is delivered and how providers themselves experience mental health in the workplace.

The term "stigma" originates from the Greek word for a mark or brand that set individuals apart, often to signal disgrace or dishonor (Goffman 1963). In the context of mental health, stigma functions as a mark of difference that devalues individuals, positioning them as less competent, less trustworthy, or less deserving of care. Sociologist Erving Goffman described stigma as a deeply discrediting attribute that reduces a person "from a whole and usual person to a tainted, discounted one." This framing remains powerful in understanding how mental health stigma operates: it is not simply about illness itself but about the social meanings imposed upon it.

Historically, mental illness has been associated with fear, misunderstanding, and exclusion (World Health Organization 2013; Rüsch et al. 2005). In many cultures, individuals with psychiatric conditions were seen as dangerous, morally weak, or even possessed, leading to their isolation in asylums or institutions. Nursing, as a profession closely tied to mental health care through its roots in asylum-based practice, has long grappled with these legacies. Early psychiatric nursing often reflected custodial approaches rather than therapeutic ones, with the primary role of nurses

N. Nami, *Unraveling Social Justice Issues in Nursing*, https://doi.org/10.1007/978-3-032-26512-8_7

being to maintain order and control. Although modern nursing has embraced holistic, patient-centered care, remnants of these historical attitudes persist, influencing how mental illness is perceived and managed today.

Despite advances in neuroscience, psychopharmacology, and psychotherapy, stigma persists across societies and healthcare systems (Thornicroft et al. 2016; World Health Organization 2013). One reason is that mental illness challenges dominant cultural values of independence, productivity, and rationality. People with mental illness may be perceived as failing to meet these ideals, resulting in marginalization. Another reason is the persistence of myths and misconceptions: that mental illness is rare, that people with psychiatric diagnoses are violent, or that conditions like depression or anxiety represent personal weakness rather than legitimate health concerns. Media portrayals often reinforce these stereotypes, shaping public perception in ways that perpetuate stigma.

The persistence of stigma also reflects structural and systemic issues (Knaak et al. 2017; World Health Organization 2013). Underfunding of mental health services, fragmentation of care, and insurance coverage limitations all signal that mental health is less valued than physical health. In many healthcare systems, mental health services remain siloed, under-resourced, and difficult to access. This institutional neglect communicates a broader cultural message: that mental health is secondary, optional, or less deserving of investment. Nurses, working within these structures, face the dual challenge of advocating for patients in a system that minimizes their needs while also navigating their own attitudes and biases.

Stigma operates at multiple levels: public stigma refers to negative stereotypes held by society at large; self-stigma occurs when individuals internalize these messages and devalue themselves; and structural stigma describes the ways in which policies and institutions perpetuate inequities (Corrigan and Watson 2002; Rüsch et al. 2005). Each of these dimensions interacts with the others, creating a reinforcing cycle that affects not only patients but also healthcare providers and systems. For example, a patient who internalizes stigma may avoid seeking care, leading to poorer outcomes, which in turn reinforces public stereotypes about the "hopelessness" of mental illness. Nurses may unconsciously absorb these societal messages, influencing their clinical decisions and the quality of care they provide.

In nursing practice, the consequences of stigma are profound (Ross and Goldner 2009; Knaak et al. 2017). Patients may withhold information about their mental health symptoms out of fear of judgment, leading to misdiagnosis or inadequate treatment. Others may delay seeking help until their conditions reach crisis points, resulting in more severe illness and greater strain on emergency and inpatient services. The therapeutic relationship, central to nursing, is undermined when patients sense even subtly that their concerns are dismissed or minimized. Addressing stigma, therefore, is not ancillary to clinical care but central to its effectiveness.

The persistence of stigma despite widespread advocacy underscores the need for a deeper, systemic response (Thornicroft et al. 2016; National Academies of Sciences, Engineering, and Medicine 2016). Anti-stigma campaigns have raised awareness, yet knowledge alone is insufficient to dismantle entrenched attitudes. What is required is cultural change within healthcare, structural reforms to elevate mental health parity, and a commitment from nurses to embody anti-stigma practices in every patient encounter. As the most trusted healthcare professionals, nurses are uniquely positioned to challenge stigma not only in their interactions with patients but also within their workplaces, communities, and professional organizations.

This chapter begins by exploring the impact of stigma on patients' experiences and health outcomes, then turns to examine how stigma manifests within nursing practice and the profession itself. It will also consider the strategies available to nurses and healthcare systems to reduce stigma, from education and advocacy to structural reforms (Thornicroft et al. 2016; Knaak et al. 2017). Ultimately, it argues that dismantling mental health stigma is inseparable from nursing's ethical mandate to advocate for dignity, justice, and holistic care.

The Impact of Stigma on Patients with Mental Health Disorders

Stigma surrounding mental illness does not merely exist as an abstract social problem; it has concrete and devastating effects on patients' health and well-being (Corrigan et al. 2014; Rüsch et al. 2005). For individuals experiencing psychiatric conditions, stigma shapes whether they seek care, how they engage with treatment, and ultimately the outcomes they achieve. The evidence consistently demonstrates that stigma functions as a barrier across the entire continuum of care from prevention to treatment to recovery producing disparities that undermine both individual health and public health goals.

One of the most significant effects of stigma is the delay or avoidance of seeking help (Corrigan et al. 2014; Henderson et al. 2013). Fear of being judged, labeled, or discriminated against often leads individuals to conceal symptoms or attempt to manage them privately. Studies show that people with depression or anxiety may wait years before seeking professional help, and for severe conditions such as schizophrenia, delays in diagnosis and treatment are common as it has been often largely visible in my area of profession as a psychiatric provider. These delays are not trivial: early intervention is strongly associated with better outcomes in nearly every mental health condition. Yet stigma fosters silence, pushing individuals into isolation and worsening their conditions before they ever encounter a nurse or provider.

Stigma also influences how patients interact with healthcare systems once they do seek care (Knaak et al. 2017; Corrigan et al. 2014). Many individuals report feeling dismissed or disbelieved when disclosing psychiatric symptoms, particularly in primary care settings where providers may attribute physical complaints to mental illness without adequate assessment a phenomenon known as diagnostic overshadowing. For example, a patient with schizophrenia who presents with chest pain may have their symptoms attributed to anxiety or psychosis, delaying appropriate cardiac workup. Such experiences not only compromise immediate health but erode trust, making patients less likely to return for future care. Nurses, who often serve as the first point of contact, are in a critical position to either reinforce or challenge these stigmatizing dynamics.

The internalization of stigma often referred to as self-stigma adds another layer of harm (Corrigan and Watson 2002; Rüsch et al. 2005). When individuals absorb society's negative messages about mental illness, they may come to view themselves as weak, incapable, or unworthy of care. This self-stigma reduces self-esteem, lowers hope for recovery, and diminishes adherence to treatment. Patients who believe their condition reflects a personal failing may resist medication, therapy, or hospitalization, fearing that acceptance of treatment confirms their "deficiency." For nurses striving to foster therapeutic relationships, counteracting self-stigma requires intentional validation, empowerment, and reinforcement of patients' strengths.

Mental health stigma also contributes to profound disparities in physical health outcomes (Knaak et al. 2017; National Academies of Sciences, Engineering, and Medicine 2016). People with serious mental illness die on average 10–20 years earlier than the general population, not only due to suicide but also to preventable physical conditions such as cardiovascular disease, diabetes, and respiratory illnesses. Stigma plays a role in this mortality gap by creating barriers to preventive care, discouraging patients from seeking treatment, and reinforcing healthcare systems that marginalize psychiatric populations. For example, individuals with severe mental illness are less likely to receive cancer screenings, vaccinations, or routine physical exams. Nurses who provide inclusive, nonjudgmental care can directly mitigate these disparities, but systemic change is necessary to fully close the gap.

The impact of stigma is magnified by its intersections with other forms of discrimination (Buettner-Schmidt and Lobo 2012; Corrigan et al. 2014). Patients of color with mental illness often face "double stigma," the combined effects of racial bias and psychiatric stigma, which further erodes access to care. Women may experience their symptoms as minimized or dismissed, reinforcing gender inequities in diagnosis and treatment. LGBTQ+ individuals, particularly transgender patients, encounter not only stigma related to mental illness but also pervasive discrimination linked to their identities, sometimes resulting in misdiagnosis or pathologization of their gender expression. Low-income individuals face additional structural barriers, with stigma compounding the disadvantages of poverty. These intersections highlight that mental health stigma cannot be understood in isolation but must be situated within broader systems of inequality.

The consequences of stigma extend beyond individual experiences to affect families and communities (Goffman 1963; Corrigan and Watson 2002). Family members of people with mental illness often experience "courtesy stigma" or "stigma by association," leading to shame, secrecy, and strained relationships. In some cultures, families may conceal a relative's condition to avoid social ostracism, delaying access to care. At the community level, stigma undermines public support for mental health services, resulting in underfunded programs, inadequate crisis response, and persistent gaps in the mental health workforce. Nurses who advocate for public health approaches to mental illness play a vital role in challenging these community-level barriers.

Stigma also contributes to a cycle of social exclusion that exacerbates the social determinants of health (Corrigan et al. 2014; World Health Organization 2013). People with psychiatric diagnoses face discrimination in employment, housing, and education, limiting their opportunities for stability and recovery. Employers may be reluctant to hire individuals with a history of mental illness, landlords may refuse housing applications, and educational institutions may fail to provide adequate support. These forms of exclusion increase poverty, homelessness, and social isolation factors that in turn worsen mental health. Nurses practicing in community and public health settings often encounter the downstream effects of these systemic barriers, reinforcing the importance of advocacy at both individual and structural levels.

Suicide is perhaps the most tragic consequence of mental health stigma (Henderson et al. 2013; Corrigan et al. 2014). Individuals experiencing suicidal thoughts often hesitate to disclose them, fearing judgment or punitive responses such as involuntary hospitalization. When stigma silences patients, opportunities for prevention are lost. Research indicates that reducing stigma increases help-seeking behavior and decreases suicidal ideation, underscoring the lifesaving importance of stigma reduction. Nurses, who frequently provide crisis intervention and suicide risk assessments, must approach such conversations with empathy, respect, and cultural humility to break through the barriers stigma creates.

The impact of stigma on patients with mental illness is multidimensional and profound (Corrigan et al. 2014; Rüsch et al. 2005). It delays diagnosis, undermines treatment, worsens health disparities, and contributes to social exclusion and early mortality. It affects not only individuals but families and communities, perpetuating cycles of disadvantage that extend far beyond the clinic walls. For nursing, these realities affirm that reducing stigma is not optional—it is central to providing effective, ethical, and equitable care.

Mental Health Stigma Within Nursing Practice

Stigma is not only experienced by patients in broader society; it also permeates the very settings where people seek healing (Ross and Goldner 2009; Schulze 2007). Healthcare, paradoxically, can both alleviate suffering and reproduce the stigma that exacerbates it. Nurses, as the largest and most trusted group of healthcare providers, are uniquely positioned to influence whether patients experience care as supportive and affirming or alienating and stigmatizing. Yet research shows that nurses, like other health professionals, are not immune to the cultural biases that surround mental illness. These biases shape clinical encounters, undermine therapeutic relationships, and contribute to persistent disparities in health outcomes.

One of the clearest ways stigma manifests in nursing practice is through attitudes toward patients with psychiatric diagnoses (Ross and Goldner 2009; Schulze 2007). Studies reveal that nurses often perceive patients with mental illness as more difficult, less compliant, or even dangerous compared to patients with physical illnesses. These perceptions can influence the quality and intensity of care provided. A patient with schizophrenia, for example, may receive less attention for their physical health concerns because providers prioritize or pathologize psychiatric symptoms. Similarly, patients with substance use disorders often classified under the umbrella of mental health conditions are frequently treated with suspicion, as though their suffering is self-inflicted or less deserving of compassion. These stigmatizing attitudes do not always arise from malice; they often reflect a lack of training, inadequate institutional support, or internalized societal stereotypes.

Diagnostic overshadowing remains a persistent problem in nursing practice (Knaak et al. 2017; Corrigan et al. 2014). When a patient with a known psychiatric history presents with new physical symptoms, there is a tendency for providers to attribute these complaints to the mental illness rather than considering alternative explanations. For instance, chest pain may be dismissed as anxiety, or lethargy as depression, delaying the diagnosis of underlying medical conditions. Nurses play a crucial role in assessment and triage, meaning their judgments can either reinforce or challenge such assumptions. When stigma drives diagnostic overshadowing, patients experience poorer outcomes and, over time, reduced trust in the healthcare system.

Stigma also shapes the therapeutic relationship, which is central to nursing practice (American Nurses Association 2020; Ross and Goldner 2009). Patients who perceive judgment, impatience, or dismissiveness from nurses are less likely to disclose sensitive information, adhere to treatment, or return for follow-up care. Even subtle cues tone of voice, body language, avoidance of eye contact can signal stigma and create distance. By contrast, when nurses actively listen, validate patients' experiences, and convey empathy, they help dismantle stigma and foster healing relationships. The difference often lies not in formal clinical interventions but in everyday practices of respect and inclusion.

Workplace cultures can amplify stigma within nursing practice (Schulze 2007; Ross and Goldner 2009). In some settings, psychiatric patients are seen as burdensome, disruptive, or even threatening, leading to an emphasis on containment rather than care. This is especially visible in emergency departments, where patients in psychiatric crisis may be triaged to the bottom of the list, restrained, or discharged without adequate follow-up. Nurses working in these environments may internalize institutional norms that prioritize efficiency and order over patient dignity. Without training in trauma-informed and recovery-oriented approaches, nurses may rely on stigmatizing practices that perpetuate cycles of mistrust between patients and providers.

The lack of integration between physical and mental healthcare further perpetuates stigma in nursing practice (Knaak et al. 2017; World Health Organization 2013). In many systems, mental health services remain siloed from general medical care, reinforcing the perception that psychiatric conditions are separate, less legitimate, or peripheral to "real" health. Nurses trained primarily in acute or physical health settings may feel ill-prepared to address psychiatric needs, defaulting to avoidance or deferral. This fragmentation not only undermines holistic care but signals to patients that their mental health is less valued. Bridging this divide requires deliberate efforts in nursing education and practice to view mental and physical health as inseparable dimensions of patient well-being.

Ethically, stigma in nursing practice presents profound challenges (American Nurses Association 2015; Buettner-Schmidt and Lobo 2012). The ANA Code of Ethics emphasizes respect for human dignity and the elimination of health disparities, yet stigmatizing attitudes contradict these commitments. When patients with mental illness are treated as less deserving of care, nursing strays from its core values. For nurses themselves, this dissonance can lead to moral distress an awareness of the right course of action but an inability to follow it due to systemic constraints or cultural pressures. Over time, moral distress erodes professional integrity, job satisfaction, and retention, particularly in high-stigma environments such as psychiatric wards or emergency departments.

It is also important to acknowledge that stigma within nursing practice is not uniform (Ross and Goldner 2009; O'Reilly et al. 2010). Attitudes vary widely depending on training, experience, and context. Nurses with specialized psychiatric training often demonstrate more positive attitudes toward patients with mental illness than those without such preparation. Exposure to patients in recovery, participation in anti-stigma education, and supportive workplace cultures can significantly reduce biases. Conversely, nurses working in resource-constrained environments with little mental health support may be more prone to frustration and stigmatizing behaviors. This variability underscores the role of education and environment in shaping stigma within practice.

Stigma within nursing practice reflects broader societal biases but has unique consequences in clinical settings (Corrigan and Watson 2002; Schulze 2007). It influences how nurses perceive patients, how they prioritize care, and how patients experience healthcare. By perpetuating diagnostic overshadowing, undermining therapeutic relationships, and reinforcing systemic inequities, stigma undermines the very principles of holistic, patient-centered care that define nursing. Recognizing and addressing stigma within practice is therefore not optional but essential for ethical, effective, and equitable nursing.

Stigma and the Nursing Workforce

While much of the discussion on mental health stigma centers on patients, it is equally important to recognize that nurses themselves are not immune to its effects (National Academies of Sciences, Engineering, and Medicine 2016; American Nurses Association 2020). In fact, stigma within the nursing workforce has become a critical but underacknowledged issue. Nurses, like all human beings, experience depression, anxiety, substance use disorders, post-traumatic stress disorder (PTSD), and other psychiatric conditions. Yet the culture of nursing and of healthcare more broadly often discourages openness about these struggles, perpetuating a climate of silence, shame, and fear of professional repercussions.

The expectation that nurses embody resilience, selflessness, and emotional stability contributes to this stigma (American Nurses Association 2020; Buettner-Schmidt and Lobo 2012). Nursing is widely perceived as a "caring profession," one in which practitioners are expected to put the needs of others above their own. While this ethos fosters dedication and compassion, it also creates unrealistic expectations that nurses should be immune to psychological distress. When nurses do struggle with mental health issues, they may perceive themselves as weak, inadequate, or unfit for practice. This internalized stigma prevents many from seeking help, even when support is urgently needed.

The demanding nature of nursing further intensifies mental health challenges (American Nurses Association 2020; QSEN Institute 2020). Nurses frequently face long shifts, staffing shortages, high patient acuity, and exposure to trauma. Burnout, moral distress, and compassion fatigue are common, particularly in high-pressure environments such as emergency departments, intensive care units, or psychiatric wards. The COVID-19 pandemic amplified these pressures, exposing nurses to unprecedented levels of stress, grief, and moral injury. Surveys conducted during the pandemic revealed alarming rates of anxiety, depression, and suicidal ideation among nurses, yet many were hesitant to disclose these struggles due to stigma and fear of career consequences.

Institutional policies and professional licensing boards often exacerbate stigma (National Academies of Sciences, Engineering, and Medicine 2016; American Nurses Association 2015). In many states, nurses are required to disclose mental health diagnoses or treatment when renewing their licenses. While intended to protect patient safety, these disclosure requirements can be punitive, deterring nurses from seeking therapy, medication, or hospitalization. The fear of losing one's license or being labeled "unfit to practice" creates a chilling effect, driving mental health concerns underground. In reality, untreated mental illness poses far greater risks than responsible treatment, yet the regulatory framework continues to reinforce stigma.

Workplace cultures can also discourage open dialogue about mental health (Schulze 2007; Ross and Goldner 2009). Nurses who admit to struggling may be met with skepticism, gossip, or diminished professional standing. Supervisors may interpret disclosures as signs of incompetence, limiting career advancement opportunities. Colleagues may distance themselves, either out of misunderstanding or discomfort. This culture of silence isolates nurses, eroding team cohesion and worsening mental health outcomes. By contrast, workplaces that normalize conversations about mental health and provide confidential support services foster resilience and reduce stigma.

Substance use disorders represent a particularly stigmatized area within nursing (National Academies of Sciences, Engineering, and Medicine 2016; Ross and Goldner 2009). Rates of substance misuse are comparable between nurses and the general population, yet when nurses struggle with addiction, the response is often punitive rather than supportive. Peer assistance programs exist in many states, offering rehabilitation and monitoring in lieu of license revocation, but participation requires disclosure, and stigma remains a major barrier. Nurses with substance use disorders may be portrayed as irresponsible or dangerous, rather than recognized as professionals with treatable illnesses. This punitive framing ignores the systemic stressors such as chronic understaffing, secondary trauma, and fatigue that contribute to substance misuse in the nursing workforce.

The stigma nurses face not only harms individuals but undermines the profession as a whole (American Nurses Association 2015; National Academies of Sciences, Engineering, and Medicine 2016). Nurses who suffer in silence are more likely to experience burnout, absenteeism, and attrition, contributing to workforce shortages that jeopardize patient care. Moral distress is magnified when nurses are unable to access mental health support, leading some to leave the profession altogether. The loss of skilled, experienced nurses is a direct consequence of stigma, with ripple effects across healthcare systems.

Efforts to address stigma within the nursing workforce must be multifaceted (Knaak et al. 2017; American Nurses Association 2020). Policy reform is essential: licensing boards must reexamine disclosure requirements to balance patient safety with the rights of nurses to seek care without fear of punishment. Workplace cultures must prioritize psychological safety, encouraging open dialogue, peer support, and access to confidential services. Nursing education must incorporate mental health literacy not only for patient care but also for self-care and professional resilience. Finally, professional organizations such as the American Nurses Association must continue to advocate for systemic change, framing mental health as an integral component of professional competence rather than a threat to it.

Ultimately, dismantling stigma within the nursing workforce is not only an ethical imperative but a practical necessity (American Nurses Association 2015; National Academies of Sciences, Engineering, and Medicine 2016). Nurses cannot provide high-quality, compassionate care to others if they are denied the same compassion and support for their own mental health. Creating a culture that values and protects the psychological well-being of nurses is central to sustaining the profession, advancing equity, and fulfilling the broader mission of healthcare.

Strategies for Reducing Stigma

The persistence of mental health stigma in nursing and healthcare underscores the need for deliberate and sustained strategies to dismantle it (Thornicroft et al. 2016; Knaak et al. 2017). Stigma does not dissolve on its own; it is maintained by cultural norms, systemic structures, and interpersonal interactions. Reducing stigma requires interventions at multiple levels, from individual nurses to healthcare institutions to broader policy frameworks. By combining education, advocacy, cultural transformation, and structural reform, nursing can play a pivotal role in reshaping how mental health is understood and addressed.

Education as a Foundation.

One of the most effective strategies for reducing stigma is education (American Association of Colleges of Nursing 2021; Knaak et al. 2017). Misconceptions about mental illness persist partly because of lack of exposure to accurate information and meaningful contact with individuals who live with psychiatric conditions. Nursing curricula must integrate robust mental health content that extends beyond symptom management to include lived experiences, recovery-oriented care, and social determinants of mental health. Simulation-based training, patient panels, and service-learning projects with mental health communities can help nursing students challenge stereotypes before they become embedded in practice. Continuing education programs for practicing nurses are equally critical, particularly in specialties where psychiatric care is less emphasized.

Contact-Based Interventions

Research consistently shows that meaningful contact with people who have lived experience of mental illness reduces stigma more effectively than education alone (Thornicroft et al. 2016; Corrigan et al. 2014). Programs that bring patients, peer specialists, and advocates into nursing classrooms and workplaces help humanize psychiatric conditions and counter stereotypes. When nurses hear firsthand accounts of resilience, recovery, and strength, they begin to view patients not as diagnoses but as individuals with agency and potential. This shift is crucial for transforming the therapeutic relationship and fostering respect in clinical encounters.

Workplace Culture Change

Reducing stigma requires creating cultures of inclusivity and psychological safety within healthcare institutions (American Nurses Association 2020; Knaak et al. 2017). Leaders must set clear expectations that discriminatory language and practices are unacceptable. Training programs on trauma-informed care, implicit bias, and cultural humility should be mandatory, not optional. Peer support programs, mentorship, and reflective practice groups can provide spaces for nurses to process their own biases and learn new approaches. Institutional policies should protect staff who disclose mental health concerns, signaling that vulnerability is not a weakness but part of professional humanity.

Integration of Mental and Physical Health

Structural stigma is reinforced when mental health is siloed from physical health (World Health Organization 2013; Knaak et al. 2017). To reduce stigma, healthcare systems must embrace integrated models of care where psychiatric and physical health services are delivered in tandem. Nurses can advocate for co-located clinics, collaborative care models, and routine mental health screening in all settings. Integration normalizes mental health as an essential component of overall health, reducing the perception that psychiatric conditions are separate, shameful, or less important.

Policy and Advocacy

At the systemic level, nurses must engage in policy advocacy to dismantle structural stigma (American Nurses Association 2015; World Health Organization 2013). This includes pushing for parity in insurance coverage for mental health services, expanding funding for community-based care, and reforming licensing requirements that penalize nurses for seeking treatment. Nurses can partner with professional organizations, advocacy groups, and legislators to amplify these efforts. By framing mental health equity as a matter of social justice, nursing advocacy can help shift policies that currently reinforce disparities.

Patient-Centered Approaches

In direct practice, nurses can adopt patient-centered approaches that explicitly counter stigma (American Nurses Association 2020; QSEN Institute 2020). This means validating patients' experiences, using respectful language, and emphasizing strengths rather than deficits. Shared decision-making, in which patients are treated as partners in their care, challenges paternalism and reinforces autonomy. Nurses should also be attentive to intersectionality, recognizing that stigma is compounded by race, gender, sexuality, socioeconomic status, and disability. By tailoring care to the unique experiences of each patient, nurses can dismantle the "one-size-fits-all" models that often perpetuate exclusion.

Evaluation and Accountability

Finally, efforts to reduce stigma must be measurable and accountable (National Academies of Sciences, Engineering, and Medicine 2016; Knaak et al. 2017). Healthcare organizations should regularly assess patients' experiences of stigma, track disparities in health outcomes, and evaluate the effectiveness of anti-stigma initiatives. Feedback from patients with lived experience should guide continuous improvement. Nurses must also engage in self-reflection and peer accountability, recognizing that stigma is not eradicated by good intentions alone but requires active, ongoing commitment.

Strategies to reduce mental health stigma must be comprehensive, sustained, and embedded across all levels of nursing and healthcare (Thornicroft et al. 2016; Knaak et al. 2017). Education, contact, workplace culture, integration of care, policy advocacy, patient-centered practice, and accountability mechanisms together create a framework for change. Nurses, by virtue of their numbers, trust, and proximity to patients, are uniquely positioned to lead these efforts. Reducing stigma is not an ancillary goal but a core responsibility of nursing, essential to fulfilling its ethical mandate of dignity, justice, and holistic care.

Toward an Anti-stigma Nursing Profession

Addressing mental health stigma in nursing is not a matter of isolated interventions or temporary campaigns; it requires a sustained transformation of professional values, institutional practices, and cultural attitudes (American Nurses Association 2015; Thornicroft et al. 2016). The work ahead involves reimagining nursing not only as a caring profession but as an anti-stigma force in healthcare and society. To achieve this, nurses must align daily practice with broader commitments to justice, dignity, and equity.

The first step is cultivating self-awareness and reflexivity among nurses (Knaak et al. 2017; Reavley and Jorm 2011). Stigma persists in part because it often operates unconsciously, shaping behaviors and assumptions without explicit intent. Nurses must engage in honest reflection about their own beliefs regarding mental illness, asking how these beliefs influence clinical interactions. Training in implicit bias, trauma-informed care, and recovery-oriented practices can equip nurses with the tools to identify and challenge internalized stigma. But self-awareness is not an endpoint; it must lead to deliberate action in the form of inclusive language, respectful communication, and equitable treatment of all patients.

Second, nursing must embrace a paradigm shift in professional culture, one that recognizes mental health as inseparable from physical health (World Health Organization 2013; American Nurses Association 2020). This requires moving beyond crisis-driven responses to psychiatric symptoms and integrating mental health into routine care across all specialties. Nurses in obstetrics, oncology, pediatrics, geriatrics, and primary care must be prepared to address mental health concerns as integral to their practice. By treating mental health as a standard component of holistic care rather than a specialized or peripheral issue, nursing can normalize conversations about mental illness and reduce stigma in everyday interactions.

Third, institutional accountability is essential (National Academies of Sciences, Engineering, and Medicine 2016; Knaak et al. 2017). Healthcare organizations cannot expect individual nurses to shoulder the burden of stigma reduction without systemic support. Institutions must provide adequate resources for mental health training, ensure equitable access to psychiatric services, and hold providers accountable for discriminatory practices. Leadership must set the tone, signaling through policy and practice that stigma has no place in care delivery. Recognition and reward systems can further incentivize anti-stigma behaviors, making them not only ethical expectations but professional standards.

Fourth, the nursing profession must extend its efforts to advocacy and policy reform (American Nurses Association 2015; World Health Organization 2013). Stigma is not confined to individual attitudes; it is embedded in structures such as licensing requirements, insurance policies, and funding priorities. Nurses, as trusted voices, are well positioned to influence these systems. Advocacy for mental health parity, expansion of community-based services, and protections for healthcare workers seeking treatment are essential steps toward dismantling structural stigma. Professional organizations, nursing unions, and academic institutions must all play active roles in advancing these policy changes.

Finally, nursing must build alliances with patients, families, and communities (Corrigan et al. 2014; Henderson et al. 2013). Stigma thrives in isolation and secrecy; it is challenged by solidarity and collective action. By partnering with people who have lived experience of mental illness, nurses can co-create models of care that reflect the values of dignity, autonomy, and recovery. Families can be engaged as allies rather than stigmatized as contributors to illness. Communities can be mobilized to demand equitable funding and inclusive services. In this broader ecosystem, nursing's advocacy can ripple outward, helping reshape cultural attitudes toward mental health beyond the walls of healthcare institutions.

The vision of an anti-stigma nursing profession is not utopian: it is practical, necessary, and achievable (American Nurses Association 2020; Knaak et al. 2017). Nurses already occupy positions of immense trust and influence. By leveraging this trust to challenge stigma, they can transform not only individual patient experiences but also systemic patterns of exclusion. The journey requires courage, persistence, and humility, but it aligns seamlessly with nursing's core mission: to advocate for dignity, to reduce suffering, and to promote health for all.

Stigma reduction must be understood as central to nursing's future (American Nurses Association 2015; Buettner-Schmidt and Lobo 2012). It is not a secondary concern but a defining feature of what it means to practice ethically and effectively. Nurses who commit to this work join a long tradition of the profession's social justice advocacy, extending the same compassion historically championed in physical care to the realm of mental health. By doing so, they move the profession closer to a vision of healthcare where no patient is diminished, no provider is silenced, and no illness is stigmatized.

References

American Association of Colleges of Nursing. The essentials: core competencies for professional nursing education. Washington, DC: AACN; 2021.

American Nurses Association. Code of ethics for nurses with interpretive statements. Silver Spring: ANA; 2015.

American Nurses Association. Nursing: scope and standards of practice. 4th ed. Silver Spring: ANA; 2020.

Buettner-Schmidt K, Lobo ML. Social justice in nursing: a review of the literature. J Adv Nurs. 2012;68(7):1486–95. https://doi.org/10.1111/j.1365-2648.2011.05884.

Corrigan PW, Watson AC. Understanding the impact of stigma on people with mental illness. World Psychiatry. 2002;1(1):16–20.

Corrigan PW, Druss BG, Perlick DA. The impact of mental illness stigma on seeking and participating in mental health care. Psychol Sci Public Interest. 2014;15(2):37–70. https://doi.org/10.1177/1529100614531398.

Goffman E. Stigma: notes on the management of spoiled identity. Englewood Cliffs: Prentice-Hall; 1963.

Henderson C, Evans-Lacko S, Thornicroft G. Mental illness stigma, help seeking, and public health programs. Am J Public Health. 2013;103(5):777–80. https://doi.org/10.2105/AJPH.2012.301056.

Knaak S, Mantler E, Szeto A. Mental illness-related stigma in healthcare: barriers to access and care and evidence-based solutions. Healthc Manage Forum. 2017;30(2):111–6. https://doi.org/10.1177/0840470416679413.

National Academies of Sciences, Engineering, and Medicine. Ending discrimination against people with mental and substance use disorders: the evidence for stigma change. Washington, DC: National Academies Press; 2016. https://doi.org/10.17226/23442.

O'Reilly CL, Bell JS, Kelly PJ, Chen TF. Exploring the relationship between mental health stigma, knowledge, and provision of pharmacy services for consumers with schizophrenia. Res Soc Adm Pharm. 2010;6(2):162–77. https://doi.org/10.1016/j.sapharm.2009.05.005.

Quality and Safety Education for Nurses (QSEN) Institute. QSEN competencies. 2020. Retrieved from http://qsen.org

Reavley NJ, Jorm AF. Stigmatizing attitudes towards people with mental disorders: findings from an Australian national survey of mental health literacy and stigma. Aust N Z J Psychiatry. 2011;45(12):1086–93. https://doi.org/10.3109/00048674.2011.621061.

Ross CA, Goldner EM. Stigma, negative attitudes and discrimination towards mental illness within the nursing profession: a review of the literature. J Psychiatr Ment Health Nurs. 2009;16(6):558–67. https://doi.org/10.1111/j.1365-2850.2009.01399.x.

Rüsch N, Angermeyer MC, Corrigan PW. Mental illness stigma: concepts, consequences, and initiatives to reduce stigma. Eur Psychiatry. 2005;20(8):529–39. https://doi.org/10.1016/j.eurpsy.2005.04.004.

Schulze B. Stigma and mental health professionals: a review of the evidence on an intricate relationship. Int Rev Psychiatry. 2007;19(2):137–55. https://doi.org/10.1080/09540260701278929.

Thornicroft G, Mehta N, Clement S, Evans-Lacko S, Doherty M, Rose D, et al. Evidence for effective interventions to reduce mental-health-related stigma and discrimination. Lancet. 2016;387(10023):1123–32. https://doi.org/10.1016/S0140-6736(15)00298-6.

World Health Organization. Mental health action plan 2013–2020. Geneva: WHO Press; 2013.

Part III

Advocacy, Practice, and Future Directions

Advocating for Change

8

Introduction: Why Advocacy Matters in Nursing

Advocacy has always been a cornerstone of the nursing profession, woven into its history, ethics, and practice (American Nurses Association 2015; Falk-Rafael 2005). At its most fundamental level, advocacy means standing up for the rights, dignity, and well-being of patients, families, and communities. It requires nurses to act not only as caregivers but as protectors, mediators, and change agents. While nurses provide direct care at the bedside, their role extends far beyond the clinical encounter. To fulfill the profession's mission of promoting health and preventing harm, nurses must address the broader systems, structures, and policies that shape health outcomes. In this way, advocacy is not a supplemental duty; it is the very heart of nursing.

Historically, nursing leaders have embodied advocacy in both practice and public life (Falk-Rafael 2005; Institute of Medicine 2011). Florence Nightingale's reform efforts during the Crimean War exemplified how nurses can change not only individual health outcomes but entire systems. Her push for sanitation, public health reforms, and evidence-based practice extended nursing's reach into the social and political domains. Similarly, nurses throughout the twentieth century championed causes such as women's suffrage, labor rights, and civil rights, showing that nursing has always been intertwined with movements for justice. Contemporary nursing advocacy builds on this legacy, tackling challenges such as healthcare disparities, systemic racism, climate change, and the rights of marginalized populations.

The ethical mandate for advocacy is clear in the profession's guiding documents (American Nurses Association 2015, 2020). The American Nurses Association's Code of Ethics states that nurses must advocate for the rights, health, and safety of patients, while also addressing broader systemic injustices. Advocacy is positioned as both an individual duty and a collective responsibility. This ethical framework makes clear that advocacy is not optional or secondary: it is integral to nursing's identity. Nurses cannot remain neutral in the face of injustice, inequity, or harm; to

N. Nami, *Unraveling Social Justice Issues in Nursing*,
https://doi.org/10.1007/978-3-032-26512-8_8

do so would betray the profession's values of compassion, justice, and respect for human dignity.

Advocacy in nursing is inseparable from social justice (Buettner-Schmidt and Lobo 2012; Falk-Rafael 2005). Health outcomes are shaped not only by biology but by the social determinants of health: access to housing, education, employment, and safe environments. Nurses encounter the effects of these inequities every day, whether through a patient who cannot afford their medications, a family struggling with food insecurity, or a community burdened by environmental toxins. These inequities are not random; they are the product of social and political structures that advantage some groups while disadvantaging others. Advocacy means recognizing these structural forces and using nursing's collective power to address them. In this way, advocacy becomes the bridge between individual care and systemic transformation.

The need for advocacy has become even more urgent in the current healthcare climate (World Health Organization 2020; National Academy of Medicine 2021). Rising costs, staffing shortages, burnout, and growing disparities threaten the sustainability of healthcare systems and the well-being of patients and providers alike. Nurses often find themselves on the front lines of these crises, witnessing firsthand the consequences of inequitable policies and inadequate resources. Advocacy offers a pathway for nurses to transform frustration into action, to channel lived experience into policy reform, and to leverage their credibility to influence decision-makers.

Importantly, advocacy operates on multiple levels (Nickitas et al. 2020; Mason et al. 2021). At the individual level, nurses advocate for patients in direct care situations, ensuring their voices are heard and their rights respected. At the organizational level, nurses push for policies that protect staff, promote safe staffing, and ensure equitable access to care. At the community and societal levels, nurses engage in legislative advocacy, public health campaigns, and grassroots movements to dismantle systemic barriers to health. This multi-level framework underscores that advocacy is not confined to boardrooms or legislatures—it is also lived out in everyday clinical practice.

The relationship between advocacy and equity deserves particular emphasis (National Academy of Medicine 2021; Buettner-Schmidt and Lobo 2012). Advocacy without equity risks reinforcing the very disparities it seeks to eliminate. For example, a nurse who advocates for one patient's access to services but fails to challenge systemic barriers that exclude entire populations may inadvertently perpetuate inequity. True advocacy requires a lens of justice, ensuring that reforms benefit not only individuals but communities, particularly those historically marginalized. Nurses must therefore embrace intersectionality in advocacy, recognizing how race, gender, disability, sexuality, and socioeconomic status intersect to shape health outcomes.

Finally, advocacy is a source of empowerment for nurses themselves (Kalb et al. 2022; Papathanasiou et al. 2014). In an era when many feel constrained by bureaucracy, documentation requirements, and productivity metrics, advocacy reclaims nursing's agency as a force for change. It reminds nurses that their voices matter, not only within the healthcare team but also in society at large. Advocacy builds solidarity, strengthens professional identity, and fosters resilience by aligning practice with purpose. It transforms nursing from a reactive profession into a proactive one, capable of shaping the future of healthcare.

Advocacy matters in nursing because it embodies the profession's core values, addresses the social determinants of health, and creates pathways for systemic change (American Nurses Association 2015; National Academy of Medicine 2021). It is an ethical mandate, a historical tradition, and a practical necessity. Nurses who advocate act not only on behalf of their patients but on behalf of justice itself, ensuring that healthcare systems reflect the dignity and humanity of all people. This introduction lays the foundation for the rest of this chapter, which will explore the many dimensions of nursing advocacy from legislative engagement to grassroots movements and chart a vision for nursing as a transformative force in society.

Legislative Advocacy in Nursing

Legislative advocacy is one of the most visible and powerful forms of nursing advocacy (Nickitas et al. 2020; Mason et al. 2021). It involves influencing laws, regulations, and public policy to improve health outcomes and ensure that healthcare systems reflect principles of justice, equity, and dignity. Nurses bring a unique and indispensable perspective to legislative processes because they stand at the intersection of policy and lived experience, seeing firsthand how laws affect patients, families, and communities. While policymakers may debate statistics and budgets, nurses witness the human consequences of policy decisions every day. This makes their voices essential in shaping legislation that truly serves the public.

Historical Foundations of Nursing Advocacy

The role of nurses in legislative advocacy has deep historical roots (Falk-Rafael 2005; Institute of Medicine 2011). Florence Nightingale herself was not only a reformer of sanitation and patient care but also a political actor who lobbied the British government for systemic reforms. In the United States, nursing pioneers such as Lillian Wald used legislative advocacy to establish school nursing programs, public health services, and child labor protections. These examples show that advocacy at the policy level has always been part of nursing's DNA. Nurses have long recognized that health cannot be separated from the conditions in which people live and that structural change requires engagement with lawmakers.

Contemporary Legislative Engagement

Today, legislative advocacy by nurses takes many forms, from lobbying Congress and state legislatures to participating in local government and advisory boards (Mason et al. 2021; Nickitas et al. 2020). Nurses advocate for issues such as safe staffing ratios, expanded access to mental health services, workplace protections, opioid crisis response, maternal health equity, and protections for vulnerable populations. Professional organizations like the American Nurses Association (ANA), National Black Nurses Association (NBNA), and National Association of School Nurses (NASN) provide platforms for collective advocacy, offering resources for nurses to engage in legislative processes. These organizations amplify the voices of individual nurses, ensuring that legislators hear not only isolated stories but the collective concerns of the profession.

Case Examples of Nurse-Led Legislative Change

There are many examples of how nurses have successfully influenced legislation (Nickitas et al. 2020; Mason et al. 2021). California's landmark nurse-to-patient staffing ratio law, passed in 1999, was the result of decades of nurse-led advocacy. The legislation improved patient outcomes, reduced nurse burnout, and set a precedent for other states. Similarly, nurses played a central role in advocating for the Mental Health Parity and Addiction Equity Act of 2008, which required insurance companies to cover mental health and substance use services at the same level as physical health services. More recently, nurses have been prominent voices in campaigns for climate change action, recognizing environmental health as a critical determinant of population health.

These case studies highlight that legislative advocacy is not abstract but results in tangible improvements for patients and communities (Mason et al. 2021; National Academy of Medicine 2021). They also illustrate how nurses can translate bedside experiences into policy reform. For example, a nurse who sees patients repeatedly admitted due to lack of affordable medications can use those stories to advocate for prescription drug reforms. Such testimony carries weight with legislators because it humanizes policy debates and connects them to real-world consequences.

Barriers to Legislative Advocacy

Despite these successes, many nurses feel unprepared or unable to engage in legislative advocacy (Papathanasiou et al. 2014; Kalb et al. 2022). Time constraints, lack of policy education, and perceptions that political engagement is outside the scope of nursing practice often serve as barriers. Some nurses fear that advocacy could jeopardize their employment or professional reputation, particularly in organizations that discourage political engagement. Others may feel overwhelmed by the complexity of legislative processes or unsure of how to translate clinical concerns into policy language.

There is also the challenge of representation (National Academy of Medicine 2021; Turale and Kunaviktikul 2019). The nursing workforce is diverse, but leadership in professional organizations and policymaking spaces often does not reflect that diversity. Ensuring that nurses from marginalized communities are represented in advocacy efforts is critical, as these voices bring unique perspectives on how policies affect populations most at risk. Legislative advocacy must therefore be inclusive and intersectional, amplifying voices that have historically been silenced in healthcare debates.

Practical Strategies for Effective Advocacy

Advocacy is often discussed in broad terms, but for nurses to make meaningful change, it must be translated into concrete strategies and actions (Nickitas et al. 2020; Mason et al. 2021). The skills required for effective advocacy are not unlike those used in clinical practice: clear communication, collaboration, assessment of evidence, and persistence in the face of obstacles. Just as nurses draw on scientific knowledge and interpersonal skill at the bedside, they must use these same tools when advancing reforms in health policy or organizational practice.

One of the most powerful tools available to nurses in advocacy is the use of storytelling (Nickitas et al. 2020; Mason et al. 2021). Legislators, administrators, and members of the public may not always grasp the intricacies of clinical language or statistical data, but they respond to human stories. When a nurse shares the experience of a patient unable to afford lifesaving medications or describes the moral distress of providing care under unsafe staffing conditions, abstract problems become personal and urgent. Storytelling humanizes health policy debates, putting faces to statistics and emotions to numbers. Importantly, nurses must learn to frame these stories within broader patterns, showing that what may appear to be an isolated incident is in fact a reflection of systemic failure.

Evidence-based data is another indispensable tool (Mason et al. 2021; Nickitas et al. 2020). While personal narratives capture attention, data provides credibility and power. Nurses can strengthen their advocacy by presenting peer-reviewed research, local health statistics, and economic analyses that demonstrate both the human and financial costs of inequitable policies. For instance, studies linking safe staffing ratios to improved patient outcomes and reduced hospital readmissions provide compelling arguments for staffing legislation. Combining evidence with lived experience ensures that advocacy is both emotionally resonant and intellectually persuasive.

Collaboration is essential in effective advocacy (Turale and Kunaviktikul 2019; Kalb et al. 2022). Nurses rarely advocate in isolation; instead, they build coalitions with colleagues, professional organizations, and interprofessional partners. Coalitions amplify voices and pool resources, making advocacy efforts more sustainable and impactful. Interdisciplinary collaboration also broadens the scope of advocacy, as physicians, social workers, psychologists, and community leaders bring complementary perspectives to shared challenges. Nurses, as trusted professionals, often serve as bridges between different groups, uniting them around common goals.

Strategic communication is another critical dimension (Mason et al. 2021; Papathanasiou et al. 2014). Advocacy requires tailoring messages to different audiences, whether testifying before a legislative committee, writing an op-ed, or presenting to hospital leadership. Nurses must learn to shift seamlessly between clinical detail and public language, ensuring clarity without oversimplification. They must also be prepared to use multiple platforms, from formal reports to social media campaigns, to reach diverse audiences. The rise of digital advocacy has created new opportunities for nurses to shape discourse in real time, whether through Twitter threads, online petitions, or virtual town halls.

Persistence is vital, as advocacy is rarely a quick process (Falk-Rafael 2005; Nickitas et al. 2020). Legislative change may take years, and institutional reform may face entrenched resistance. Nurses must view advocacy as an ongoing commitment rather than a one-time event. Success often requires sustained engagement, follow-up with decision-makers, and adaptation of strategies when initial efforts do not succeed. Just as nurses persist in caring for patients through setbacks, they must also persist in advocacy, trusting that cumulative efforts will eventually yield progress.

Finally, advocacy is strengthened by preparation and mentorship (Kalb et al. 2022; AACN 2021). Nurses who are new to advocacy may feel intimidated by the complexity of political and institutional systems. Training programs, mentorship networks, and professional organizations provide guidance, demystifying processes and offering practical tools. Experienced nurse advocates play a crucial role in mentoring the next generation, passing on strategies, lessons, and encouragement. This intergenerational transfer of knowledge ensures that advocacy does not depend on individual champions alone but becomes a sustained professional tradition.

Together, these strategies, storytelling, evidence-based data, collaboration, strategic communication, persistence, and mentorship, equip nurses to be effective advocates (Nickitas et al. 2020; Mason et al. 2021). Advocacy is not an abstract concept but a skillset that can be cultivated, refined, and applied across settings. When these strategies are used in combination, they magnify each other's impact, making nurses powerful agents of systemic change.

Education, Empowerment, and Grassroots Movements in Nursing Advocacy

Advocacy in nursing does not occur by accident; it must be cultivated intentionally through education, empowerment, and the building of collective movements (AACN 2021; Kalb et al. 2022). Nurses cannot be expected to become effective advocates if they are not provided with the knowledge, skills, and confidence to speak up on behalf of patients, colleagues, and communities. Education, both in academic settings and through ongoing professional development, plays a critical role in shaping the next generation of nurse advocates. Nursing schools that integrate advocacy into curricula prepare students to see themselves not only as clinicians but as social change agents. Courses that connect health policy, social determinants of health, and leadership skills encourage students to link their daily practice with larger systemic concerns. Clinical placements in community-based settings or with advocacy organizations expose students to real-world inequities and demonstrate how nurses can intervene beyond the hospital walls.

The emphasis on empowerment is equally critical (Kalb et al. 2022; Sigma Theta Tau International 2020). Many nurses, particularly those early in their careers or working in marginalized communities, may feel powerless in the face of large systems and entrenched hierarchies. Empowerment comes when nurses recognize that their voices carry authority, not only because of their expertise but because of the trust society places in them. Professional organizations reinforce this empowerment by providing mentorship, resources, and opportunities for direct engagement in advocacy. When nurses see colleagues successfully influencing policy or leading community initiatives, they begin to envision themselves as capable of doing the same. Empowerment also comes from solidarity. When nurses act collectively rather than individually, their power multiplies. Speaking out as a unified group not only amplifies the message but also provides protection and encouragement to those who may otherwise hesitate to raise their voices.

Grassroots movements in nursing demonstrate the power of collective action (Falk-Rafael 2005; APHA 2019). History is filled with examples of nurses banding together to advocate for issues ranging from labor rights to public health reforms. Contemporary movements continue this tradition. Nurse-led organizations have mobilized around racial equity, climate change, gun violence prevention, and the opioid epidemic. These grassroots efforts are powerful precisely because they emerge from the lived realities of nursing practice, giving them authenticity and urgency. For instance, when nurses spoke out during the height of the COVID-19 pandemic about unsafe working conditions and lack of protective equipment, they did so not as distant observers but as frontline witnesses. Their advocacy drew national attention and shaped public discourse about the responsibilities of health systems and governments to protect healthcare workers.

Grassroots advocacy is also increasingly supported by digital platforms (World Health Organization 2020; Mason et al. 2021). Social media has become a powerful tool for nurses to organize, share stories, and mobilize action. Hashtags, online petitions, and virtual campaigns can spread rapidly, reaching audiences far beyond traditional professional networks. This form of digital activism is particularly important for younger nurses, who are often more comfortable navigating these spaces and who bring fresh perspectives to advocacy. Yet the digital sphere also requires careful navigation, as professionalism, privacy, and credibility must be maintained even while pushing for bold change.

Education, empowerment, and grassroots organizing are not isolated from one another; they reinforce each other (Kalb et al. 2022; AACN 2021). Education lays the groundwork, equipping nurses with the knowledge and frameworks to understand inequities. Empowerment gives them the confidence to act. Grassroots movements provide the structure and solidarity to turn individual efforts into systemic change. When these elements align, nursing advocacy becomes not just reactive but transformative, capable of reshaping healthcare systems and influencing broader social policies.

This dynamic interplay points to the necessity of seeing advocacy not as an optional add-on to nursing practice but as a skillset to be nurtured from the beginning of professional formation (AACN 2021; American Nurses Association 2015). Just as nurses are trained to interpret lab results or administer medications, they must also be trained to identify inequities, craft persuasive arguments, and mobilize collective action. Without this foundation, the profession risks leaving its advocacy potential unrealized. With it, nurses are prepared to not only care for individuals but also to challenge the structures that produce illness and inequity in the first place.

The Future of Nursing Advocacy

The future of nursing advocacy lies in its ability to adapt to emerging challenges while remaining rooted in the profession's enduring values of compassion, justice, and respect for human dignity (American Nurses Association 2015; World Health Organization 2020). As healthcare continues to evolve in response to demographic shifts, technological innovation, and global crises, nurses must expand their advocacy beyond traditional boundaries and embrace new avenues for change. The next generation of nurse advocates will need to think not only locally or nationally but globally, recognizing that health inequities are interconnected across borders. Climate change, pandemics, migration, and the globalization of healthcare systems all require collaborative approaches that transcend individual institutions or countries. Nurses, with their presence in nearly every part of the world, are uniquely positioned to act as global advocates, uniting across cultures to demand policies that protect the health of people and the planet.

International organizations such as the World Health Organization and the International Council of Nurses already provide frameworks for global advocacy, but grassroots nurse-led movements will continue to drive much of the momentum (World Health Organization 2020; Turale and Kunaviktikul 2019). Campaigns for universal health coverage, access to vaccines, and responses to humanitarian crises demonstrate how nurses can amplify global health agendas while drawing on local expertise. At the same time, nurses must push for recognition of their own professional rights on the world stage, ensuring that they are supported and protected in the often-dangerous environments in which they work. Global advocacy also calls for solidarity across borders, where nurses from resource-rich countries partner with colleagues in resource-limited settings to share knowledge, strengthen infrastructure, and build equitable health systems.

Digital tools will increasingly shape the landscape of advocacy (Mason et al. 2021; Sigma Theta Tau International 2020). The expansion of social media, online networks, and digital communication platforms has already transformed how nurses organize, educate, and mobilize. Digital advocacy allows for rapid dissemination of information, direct engagement with policymakers, and the ability to reach audiences previously inaccessible. Hashtags, webinars, podcasts, and virtual town halls are no longer fringe activities but integral strategies for raising awareness and influencing change. For nurses, this means embracing digital literacy as a professional competency, ensuring that they can use technology not only for clinical practice but also for advocacy. At the same time, digital spaces must be navigated carefully, with attention to credibility, professionalism, and privacy. The challenge for the future will be to harness the power of digital advocacy while maintaining the trust that has long been nursing's greatest asset.

The vision of equity-centered nursing advocacy must also continue to evolve (National Academy of Medicine 2021; APHA 2019). Nurses must ensure that advocacy efforts address not only immediate patient needs but also the structural determinants of health that perpetuate inequities. This requires adopting intersectional frameworks that acknowledge the overlapping influences of race, gender, socioeconomic status, disability, and sexual orientation. Advocacy that fails to recognize these intersections risks reinforcing disparities rather than dismantling them. The future of advocacy will be measured not simply by the number of laws passed or policies changed but by the tangible reduction in health inequities and the improvement of outcomes for those who have historically been marginalized.

Another critical direction lies in preparing the nursing workforce itself to embrace advocacy as an essential component of professional practice (AACN 2021; Kalb et al. 2022). Nursing education must continue to evolve, embedding advocacy into curricula as a core competency rather than an elective topic. Students must be taught not only the technical skills of advocacy such as policy analysis, persuasive communication, and coalition building but also the ethical imperative that drives it. Faculty and mentors must model advocacy in action, showing students how to balance bedside care with systemic engagement. Without this deliberate preparation, advocacy risks being seen as peripheral rather than central to nursing identity.

Finally, the future of advocacy will require resilience and creativity (Falk-Rafael 2005; Kalb et al. 2022). Nurses will face resistance, whether from entrenched power structures, political opposition, or institutional inertia. Advocacy efforts may not always succeed immediately, and progress will often come in incremental steps. Yet resilience, the ability to persist despite setbacks, will sustain the profession's efforts. Creativity will also be essential, as nurses will need to find innovative solutions to complex problems, drawing on research, technology, and community partnerships. By combining resilience and creativity with the profession's deep-rooted commitment to justice, nursing can shape a future in which advocacy is not a side role, but an integral thread woven into the very fabric of healthcare.

Advocating for change in nursing is about more than influencing individual policies or institutions (National Academy of Medicine 2021; Nickitas et al. 2020). It is about shaping a profession that sees itself as a force for equity and justice in a world where health is increasingly shaped by global, structural, and systemic forces. Nurses are not only caregivers; they are leaders, change agents, and advocates whose voices carry immense power. By embracing advocacy as a professional obligation and a source of empowerment, nurses can continue to transform not only the systems in which they work but the very societies they serve. The work is challenging and ongoing, but the vision is clear: a nursing profession that speaks boldly, acts justly, and advocates relentlessly for a healthier and more equitable world.

References

American Association of Colleges of Nursing. The essentials: core competencies for professional nursing education. AACN; 2021.

American Nurses Association. Code of ethics for nurses with interpretive statements. ANA; 2015.

American Nurses Association. Nursing: scope and standards of practice. 4th ed. ANA; 2020.

American Public Health Association. Nursing's role in addressing discrimination: protecting and promoting health for all. APHA Policy Statement; 2019.

Buettner-Schmidt K, Lobo ML. Social justice in nursing: a review of the literature. J Adv Nurs. 2012;68(7):1446–57. https://doi.org/10.1111/j.1365-2648.2011.05884.x.

Falk-Rafael A. Speaking truth to power: nursing's legacy and moral imperative. Adv Nurs Sci. 2005;28(3):212–23.

Institute of Medicine. The future of nursing: leading change, advancing health. National Academies Press; 2011.

Kalb KA, O'Conner F, Watson C. Building advocacy capacity in nursing: the role of leadership and mentorship. J Nurs Manag. 2022;30(2):249–58. https://doi.org/10.1111/jonm.13372.

Mason DJ, Perez A, McLemore MR. Policy and political competence of nurses: advancing the agenda. J Nurs Scholarsh. 2021;53(2):131–40. https://doi.org/10.1111/jnu.12628.

National Academy of Medicine. The future of nursing 2020–2030: charting a path to achieve health equity. National Academies Press; 2021. https://doi.org/10.17226/25982.

Nickitas DM, Middaugh DJ, Aries N. Policy and politics for nurses and other health professionals: advocacy and action. 3rd ed. Jones & Bartlett; 2020.

Papathanasiou IV, Tsaras K, Sarafis P. Views and perceptions of nursing students on their role in the health care system and society. Int J Health Policy Manag. 2014;3(2):91–4. https://doi.org/10.15171/ijhpm.2014.63.

Sigma Theta Tau International. Nurses leading change: advancing health through advocacy. Sigma; 2020.

Turale S, Kunaviktikul W. The contribution of nurses to health policy and advocacy requires leadership, global collaboration, and political competence. Int Nurs Rev. 2019;66(3):302–4. https://doi.org/10.1111/inr.12550.

World Health Organization. State of the world's nursing 2020: investing in education, jobs and leadership. WHO; 2020.

Advocating for Independence of Nurse Practitioners in the United States

9

The Role of Nurse Practitioners (NPs) in the United States

The role of nurse practitioners (NPs) in the United States has grown dramatically since the position first emerged in the mid-1960s, born out of necessity to meet gaps in primary care, especially for children and underserved populations (Lugo et al. 2007; Institute of Medicine 2011). Initially envisioned as a collaborative extension of nursing practice, the NP role quickly evolved into one of the most transformative forces in modern healthcare. Today, more than 355,000 licensed nurse practitioners provide care across diverse settings in the United States, and the demand for their expertise continues to increase in response to physician shortages, the aging population, and the complex needs of communities. Despite their proven effectiveness and the advanced training they undergo—graduate-level education, national certification, and extensive clinical preparation—NPs still face significant restrictions on their scope of practice in many states. This tension between training and autonomy lies at the heart of ongoing advocacy efforts for full practice authority.

Advocating for independence does not mean positioning nurse practitioners in opposition to physicians or other health professionals (National Academy of Medicine 2021; American Nurses Association 2021). Rather, it is about aligning scope of practice laws with the competencies of NPs and the pressing needs of patients. Full practice authority (FPA) allows NPs to evaluate patients, diagnose conditions, interpret diagnostic tests, and initiate treatment plans including prescribing medications without mandatory physician oversight. In practice, most NPs already perform these functions, but in states without FPA, they must do so under a written agreement with a physician, even when that collaboration is largely administrative rather than clinical. This creates unnecessary barriers that delay care, inflate costs, and undermine the efficiency of the healthcare system.

The importance of advocating for NP independence cannot be overstated (American Association of Nurse Practitioners 2022; National Academy of Medicine 2021). The United States faces a looming primary care crisis, with estimates

N. Nami, *Unraveling Social Justice Issues in Nursing*, https://doi.org/10.1007/978-3-032-26512-8_9

projecting a shortage of up to 48,000 primary care physicians by 2034. Rural areas, in particular, bear the brunt of this shortage, as fewer physicians choose to practice in isolated communities where resources are scarce. Nurse practitioners have repeatedly proven their ability to fill these gaps, offering high-quality, cost-effective, and patient-centered care. Studies consistently demonstrate that NP outcomes in primary care are equivalent to, and in some cases exceed, those of physicians, particularly in patient satisfaction, preventive services, and chronic disease management. Restricting their practice not only wastes a highly skilled workforce but exacerbates inequities in access to care.

The ethical dimension of this issue also deserves emphasis (American Nurses Association 2015; Buettner-Schmidt and Lobo 2012). Nursing has long grounded itself in the principles of advocacy, equity, and justice. Denying NPs the ability to practice to the full extent of their training is not simply a professional issue: it is a social justice issue. Communities already disadvantaged by poverty, geography, or systemic inequities are disproportionately harmed by restrictive practice laws. Patients in these communities may wait weeks for appointments, travel hours to see a provider, or forgo care altogether. Granting NPs full practice authority is, therefore, a matter of equity: ensuring that all individuals, regardless of where they live or their socioeconomic background, have timely access to competent, compassionate care.

At the same time, advocacy for NP independence raises important questions about hierarchy and power within healthcare (Buettner-Schmidt and Lobo 2012; National Academy of Medicine 2021). Physicians have traditionally held dominant authority in the system, reinforced by historical, cultural, and political structures. The push for NP independence challenges this hierarchy by asserting that other providers are equally capable of leading in primary care and beyond. This is not an attack on the medical profession but an acknowledgment of the collaborative reality of modern healthcare. Advocacy must balance respect for interprofessional collaboration with the recognition that arbitrary restrictions harm patients and communities.

Globally, the United States lags behind many nations in granting independence to nurse practitioners and advanced practice nurses (World Health Organization 2020; National Academy of Medicine 2021). Countries such as Canada, the United Kingdom, and Australia have implemented models where NPs practice autonomously, supported by robust regulatory frameworks. These models demonstrate that autonomy does not compromise safety or quality but strengthens health systems by expanding access and reducing bottlenecks. The United States, with its fragmented state-by-state approach, leaves NPs subject to a patchwork of laws that vary widely, creating confusion and limiting mobility within the profession. For example, an NP practicing independently in Arizona may move to Texas and suddenly find themselves unable to prescribe medication without physician sign-off. Such inconsistencies highlight the urgent need for federal-level reforms to standardize NP practice authority.

The COVID-19 pandemic underscored the critical role of NPs in responding to public health crises and exposed the inefficiencies of restrictive practice laws (World

Health Organization 2020; Phillips 2022). During the emergency, many states temporarily suspended physician oversight requirements, allowing NPs to practice more freely to meet urgent demands. These temporary measures demonstrated what has long been known: nurse practitioners can provide safe, effective, and independent care without unnecessary supervision. The outcomes of these temporary waivers provided a natural experiment that bolsters the case for permanent reform. Yet as the pandemic waned, many states reverted to restrictive practices, revealing the entrenched resistance to structural change. Advocacy, therefore, must not only highlight evidence but also sustain pressure to translate temporary gains into permanent policy.

At its core, the advocacy for NP independence reflects a broader transformation in how the United States conceptualizes healthcare delivery (National Academy of Medicine 2021; Institute of Medicine 2011). It calls for a move away from physician-centric models toward team-based, patient-centered systems that leverage the full talents of all professionals. It requires dismantling outdated hierarchies and replacing them with systems that prioritize equity, efficiency, and access. For nurse practitioners, independence is not a privilege to be granted by the medical establishment but a recognition of their training, competence, and contributions to healthcare. For patients, NP independence is a pathway to more accessible, affordable, and timely care.

This chapter will explore the historical, political, and ethical dimensions of NP independence, examine the barriers that continue to impede progress, and present strategies for effective advocacy. It will highlight case studies from states that have already embraced full practice authority, drawing lessons from their successes and challenges (Phillips 2022; American Association of Nurse Practitioners 2022). It will also situate NP advocacy within global contexts, comparing the United States to other healthcare systems where nurse autonomy is fully realized. Ultimately, the argument is clear: advocating for NP independence is not only about advancing the nursing profession but about ensuring that patients receive the care they deserve in a healthcare system that works for all.

Historical and Policy Context of NP Practice

The origins of the nurse practitioner role can be traced to the mid-1960s, a period when the United States was experiencing significant shortages in primary care, particularly in pediatrics and family medicine (Lugo et al. 2007; Institute of Medicine 2011). Dr. Loretta Ford, a nurse, and Dr. Henry Silver, a physician, created the first nurse practitioner program at the University of Colorado in 1965. Their vision was to expand the capabilities of nurses through advanced clinical education, equipping them to provide preventive and primary care services at a time when large segments of the population lacked reliable access to physicians. The program proved successful, and similar educational models spread rapidly across the country. By the 1970s, nurse practitioners were beginning to be recognized as a crucial component of the healthcare workforce.

From the outset, however, the role of the nurse practitioner was defined within the context of medical authority (Lugo et al. 2007; Institute of Medicine 2011). Scope-of-practice laws regulations that determine what healthcare providers are legally permitted to do were initially framed around the assumption that physicians held ultimate oversight. Nurse practitioners were required to work under "collaborative agreements" with physicians, agreements that often dictated their ability to prescribe medications, order diagnostic tests, or establish treatment plans. While some collaborations were functional partnerships that enhanced care delivery, many were purely administrative, existing to satisfy legal requirements rather than clinical need.

Over time, the debate over scope of practice intensified (Phillips 2022; Xue et al. 2016). Advocates argued that NPs were being held back by outdated regulatory structures that did not reflect their training or competence. Opponents, primarily physician groups such as the American Medical Association (AMA), contended that physician oversight was necessary to ensure safety and quality of care. This debate became deeply political, playing out in state legislatures where scope-of-practice laws are determined. Because there is no single federal standard, the United States has developed a patchwork system in which NP authority varies dramatically depending on the state.

Today, this patchwork can be divided into three categories: full practice authority, reduced practice, and restricted practice (American Association of Nurse Practitioners 2022; Phillips 2022). In states with full practice authority, NPs can evaluate patients, diagnose, order and interpret tests, and prescribe independently. As of 2023, 27 states, the District of Columbia, and two US territories grant full practice authority. In reduced practice states, NPs may practice independently in some areas but must maintain a collaborative agreement with a physician for certain functions, such as prescribing controlled substances. In restricted practice states, physician oversight is required for nearly all aspects of care, limiting NPs' ability to practice autonomously. This inconsistency creates barriers to mobility and prevents nurse practitioners from contributing fully to addressing nationwide shortages.

The evolution of these laws has been shaped not only by debates over clinical competence but by power dynamics within healthcare (Buettner-Schmidt and Lobo 2012; Phillips 2022). Physician organizations have historically wielded significant influence in state legislatures, lobbying to maintain supervisory requirements. Meanwhile, nursing organizations such as the American Association of Nurse Practitioners (AANP) and the American Nurses Association (ANA) have fought to expand authority, presenting evidence that NPs deliver safe, effective, and cost-efficient care. The clash between these groups has often slowed reform, even when data overwhelmingly supports NP independence.

Federal policy has also played a role, though indirectly (National Academy of Medicine 2021; National Council of State Boards of Nursing 2017). Medicare and Medicaid reimbursement policies have historically mirrored state-level restrictions, reimbursing NPs at lower rates than physicians for the same services or requiring physician co-signature for billing. While some progress has been made in equalizing reimbursement, disparities persist, reinforcing structural inequities in recognition and compensation. Furthermore, national agencies have often deferred to state boards of nursing and medicine, perpetuating the fragmented regulatory environment.

The historical trajectory of NP practice authority illustrates how social, cultural, and political forces intersect with healthcare delivery (Institute of Medicine 2011; Buettner-Schmidt and Lobo 2012). On the one hand, the creation of the NP role was a groundbreaking innovation that expanded access to care and redefined nursing practice. On the other hand, the enduring restrictions on NP authority reveal the persistence of hierarchical thinking in healthcare, where physician dominance is preserved through legal and regulatory frameworks. These tensions have produced a system in which patient access depends as much on geography and politics as on professional competence.

The pandemic of 2020 provided a dramatic example of how policy can shift under pressure (Phillips 2022; World Health Organization 2020). As the healthcare system strained under the weight of COVID-19, several states temporarily lifted restrictions on NP practice, recognizing the urgent need for every available provider. These waivers demonstrated that nurse practitioners could practice safely and effectively without mandated physician oversight, even in high-stakes environments. Yet when the emergency subsided, many states reinstated restrictions, underscoring the political, rather than clinical, nature of scope-of-practice debates. The experience also galvanized advocacy efforts, providing concrete evidence that restrictions are unnecessary barriers to care.

Understanding this historical and policy context is essential for advocacy (Nickitas et al. 2020; American Association of Nurse Practitioners 2022). It highlights that the fight for NP independence is not just about clinical evidence but about challenging entrenched power structures and political influence. Advocates must be prepared to address not only questions of safety and quality but also the broader dynamics of professional hierarchies, legislative lobbying, and public perception. The history of NP practice authority demonstrates that progress is possible, half the states have embraced full practice authority, but also that advocacy must be persistent, strategic, and grounded in both data and ethical arguments.

Barriers to NP Practice

Despite decades of evidence demonstrating the safety, quality, and cost-effectiveness of nurse practitioner care, the road toward independence remains obstructed by multiple barriers (Poghosyan et al. 2017; Xue et al. 2016). These barriers are not primarily clinical; rather, they are rooted in politics, economics, and deeply embedded hierarchies within the healthcare system. Understanding the nature of these barriers is crucial for designing effective advocacy strategies, as each reflects not only professional tensions but also broader cultural assumptions about authority, expertise, and equity in healthcare.

Perhaps the most significant barrier is organized physician opposition (Phillips 2022; American Association of Nurse Practitioners 2022). Groups such as the

American Medical Association and state medical societies have long resisted efforts to expand NP scope of practice, often framing their arguments in terms of patient safety. While patient safety is a legitimate concern in any discussion of healthcare reform, this framing frequently ignores the robust evidence base confirming that nurse practitioners provide care that is equivalent to physicians in quality and outcomes. Systematic reviews, meta-analyses, and decades of research show no significant differences in mortality, hospitalization, or complication rates when care is delivered by NPs compared to physicians. Yet opponents continue to argue that physician supervision is necessary, a position that reflects less about the evidence and more about professional turf. In many cases, resistance is tied to maintaining control over healthcare delivery and protecting physician dominance within the system.

Lobbying plays a central role in sustaining restrictive policies (Phillips 2022; American Nurses Association 2021). Physician organizations wield significant financial and political influence at both state and federal levels. They contribute to campaigns, mobilize their memberships, and maintain longstanding relationships with lawmakers. In contrast, nursing organizations historically have fewer financial resources and less political clout, though this imbalance has begun to shift in recent years. The result has been uneven progress: some states have embraced full practice authority, while others remain entrenched in restrictive frameworks. The political dynamics often outweigh the clinical evidence, leaving policy shaped by influence rather than by patient needs.

Reimbursement inequities form another significant barrier (Poghosyan et al. 2017; National Academy of Medicine 2021). Even in states with full practice authority, NPs are often reimbursed at lower rates than physicians for the same services. Medicare, for example, reimburses NPs at 85% of the physician fee schedule, despite evidence showing the quality of care is comparable. Private insurers frequently mirror these reimbursement structures, further entrenching inequities. Lower reimbursement not only undermines NP independence but also limits the financial sustainability of NP-led practices. It signals a systemic undervaluing of NP contributions, reinforcing the perception that their work is somehow less valuable than that of physicians.

Structural bias and hierarchical culture within healthcare also constrain NP independence (Buettner-Schmidt and Lobo 2012; National Academy of Medicine 2021). The medical profession has historically occupied the pinnacle of healthcare authority, and even when NPs demonstrate expertise, they are often perceived through the lens of subordination. This dynamic is particularly pronounced in hospital systems and academic medical centers, where rigid hierarchies persist. The language of "mid-level providers" or "physician extenders" further marginalizes NPs, reducing their role to that of helpers rather than independent professionals. Such terminology is not neutral; it reflects and reinforces cultural assumptions that undermine NP autonomy.

Geographic and political disparities exacerbate these barriers (Kuo et al. 2013; Phillips 2022). Because scope-of-practice laws are determined at the state level, NPs face very different realities depending on where they work. In one state, an NP may establish an independent primary care clinic, while in another, they cannot prescribe basic medications without a physician's signature. This inconsistency undermines mobility within the profession and creates confusion for patients and providers alike. It also perpetuates inequities in access, as states with the greatest healthcare shortages often maintain the most restrictive laws.

These barriers also intersect with issues of race, gender, and power (Buettner-Schmidt and Lobo 2012; National Academy of Medicine 2021). The majority of nurse practitioners are women, and nursing has historically been devalued as a female-dominated profession. The resistance to NP independence cannot be disentangled from this broader history of gendered hierarchies in healthcare. Physician dominance, reinforced by lobbying and institutional structures, reflects not only professional self-interest but also patriarchal norms that have long privileged medicine over nursing. For nurse practitioners of color, these dynamics are compounded by racial inequities, further marginalizing their authority and limiting their influence in policy debates.

The persistence of these barriers has profound implications for patients (Xue et al. 2016; Kuo et al. 2013). Restrictive practice laws delay care, limit access, and drive up costs. They perpetuate healthcare inequities by concentrating authority in a profession that is less diverse and less equitably distributed than nursing. They also undermine the morale of NPs, many of whom report frustration at being unable to practice to the full extent of their training. This frustration contributes to workforce shortages, as talented clinicians leave states with restrictive laws for those with greater autonomy, exacerbating disparities in access.

Taken together, these barriers underscore the reality that advocacy for NP independence is not simply about presenting clinical evidence but about confronting entrenched power structures (Buettner-Schmidt and Lobo 2012; Phillips 2022). Overcoming them will require political engagement, coalition building, and cultural change within healthcare. It will require reframing the conversation from one about professional turf to one about patient access and equity. As the history of NP advocacy shows, progress is possible but only when barriers are identified clearly and addressed strategically.

Impact of Restrictive Practice Laws

The consequences of restrictive practice laws extend far beyond professional disputes between nursing and medicine; they have a direct and measurable impact on patients, communities, healthcare costs, and the overall strength of the US healthcare system (Xue et al. 2016; Kuo et al. 2013). While opponents of nurse practitioner independence often frame these restrictions as protective measures, the evidence shows that they function instead as barriers that undermine access to care, worsen health inequities, and contribute to systemic inefficiencies.

For patients, restrictive practice laws translate into fewer available providers, longer wait times, and delays in diagnosis and treatment (Kuo et al. 2013; Xue et al. 2016). In states where NPs face limitations, patients in rural or underserved areas often experience the most severe consequences. Rural communities already face critical shortages of primary care providers, with many counties designated as health professional shortage areas by the Health Resources and Services Administration (HRSA). Nurse practitioners are more likely than physicians to practice in these areas, yet restrictions force them to maintain costly and sometimes unnecessary supervisory agreements with physicians who may not even reside locally. This creates bottlenecks that delay essential care and in some cases forces patients to forgo treatment altogether. The result is a perpetuation of health disparities that disproportionately harm populations already marginalized by geography, poverty, or race.

The cost of healthcare is another area profoundly affected by restrictive laws (Poghosyan et al. 2017; Xue et al. 2016). Studies consistently show that care delivered by nurse practitioners is cost-effective, both for patients and for the system as a whole. NPs emphasize preventive care and chronic disease management, areas that reduce hospitalizations and emergency department visits when done effectively. Yet requiring physician oversight increases administrative costs and duplicates services without improving outcomes. Patients may be billed twice, once for the NP and again for the physician who signs off, even if the physician has had no direct involvement in the care. From a systems perspective, this inefficiency drives up healthcare spending while offering no added value. Expanding NP independence could help reduce costs in a system already burdened by unsustainable expenditures.

Restrictive practice also affects patient choice and satisfaction (Poghosyan et al. 2017; American Association of Nurse Practitioners 2023). In many communities, NPs are the most accessible providers, and patients often report high levels of satisfaction with NP care. Research shows that patients appreciate the time, communication, and holistic approach that NPs bring to clinical encounters. However, restrictions limit the ability of NPs to establish independent clinics or expand services, thereby constraining patient choice. In effect, patients are denied the opportunity to select the provider they trust most, not because of quality concerns but because of outdated regulations.

The workforce implications are equally significant (National Council of State Boards of Nursing 2017; Kuo et al. 2013). Restrictive practice laws contribute to uneven distribution of healthcare providers across the country. NPs who might otherwise practice in restrictive states may relocate to those with full practice authority, leading to workforce imbalances. This "brain drain" effect further exacerbates shortages in states that most need expanded access. Moreover, restrictions can discourage new graduates from entering underserved markets, as the cost and burden of maintaining supervisory agreements make independent practice financially unfeasible. Over time, this contributes to burnout, attrition, and reduced morale among NPs, undermining the sustainability of the workforce.

Restrictive policies also hinder innovation in healthcare delivery (National Academy of Medicine 2021; World Health Organization 2020). In states with full practice authority, NPs have pioneered models of care such as NP-led clinics, telehealth services, and integrated community health programs. These models expand access, particularly for vulnerable populations, and demonstrate the flexibility and creativity of the nursing profession. By contrast, restrictive states stifle such innovation, as regulatory barriers limit the ability of NPs to experiment with new approaches. The result is a two-tiered system in which some states reap the benefits of modern, nurse-driven care models while others remain locked in outdated frameworks.

From an equity perspective, the harms of restrictive practice laws are especially concerning (Buettner-Schmidt and Lobo 2012; National Academy of Medicine 2021). Communities of color, rural populations, and low-income groups bear the brunt of limited access. Many of these communities rely heavily on nurse practitioners as their primary providers, yet the barriers prevent them from receiving timely, comprehensive care. Restrictive practice laws thus perpetuate existing inequities in healthcare delivery, widening the gap between those who can access care easily and those who cannot. Advocacy for NP independence, therefore, must be understood not only as a professional issue but also as an equity and justice issue.

The cumulative impact of these restrictions undermines the very goals of the healthcare system: to provide safe, efficient, equitable, and accessible care (National Academy of Medicine 2021; World Health Organization 2020). By artificially limiting the ability of a highly trained workforce to contribute fully, restrictive practice laws waste valuable resources and exacerbate shortages. They harm patients directly, increase costs unnecessarily, and weaken the resilience of the healthcare system as a whole. The evidence is overwhelming that independence for nurse practitioners benefits patients, communities, and systems alike, while restrictions serve only to protect entrenched hierarchies.

Advocacy Strategies

If restrictive practice laws persist not because of evidence but because of entrenched power dynamics, then advocacy for nurse practitioner independence must be strategic, sustained, and multifaceted (Phillips 2022; American Nurses Association 2021). Advocacy in this domain cannot rely solely on clinical data, though evidence remains a critical component. It must also encompass legislative action, coalition building, public engagement, and the cultivation of leadership within the profession. Nurse practitioners, as trusted voices in healthcare, hold both the credibility and the lived experience necessary to drive change, but their efforts are most effective when organized and amplified through collective action.

Legislative advocacy remains the cornerstone of the movement for full practice authority (American Association of Nurse Practitioners 2022; Phillips 2022). Because scope-of-practice laws are determined at the state level, NPs must engage directly with state legislatures, where decisions about independence are debated and codified. This requires more than submitting testimony; it requires building relationships with lawmakers, educating them about the realities of patient care, and countering misinformation spread by opposing groups. Legislators often lack familiarity with the intricacies of healthcare delivery, and they may rely heavily on input from physicians, who have historically held greater political sway. For this reason, nurse practitioners must develop the skills to translate their experiences into persuasive arguments that resonate with policymakers. Telling the story of a rural community that lost access to primary care because an NP could not maintain a supervisory agreement is often more compelling than statistics alone. Advocacy is as much about narrative as it is about numbers.

Coalition building is equally critical (American Nurses Association 2021; National Academy of Medicine 2021). Nurses rarely achieve legislative victories in isolation. Successful campaigns often bring together diverse stakeholders who share common goals, such as expanding access to care and reducing costs. Patient advocacy groups, rural health associations, public health organizations, and even some forward-thinking physician allies can serve as powerful partners. These coalitions broaden the base of support, framing NP independence not as a nursing issue but as a community issue. The inclusion of patients' voices is particularly impactful. When patients speak about the difficulty of accessing care under restrictive laws, lawmakers are forced to confront the human consequences of policy inertia.

Evidence-based advocacy provides the backbone for these efforts (Poghosyan et al. 2017; Xue et al. 2016). A robust body of research confirms that nurse practitioners deliver high-quality, safe, and effective care. Decades of studies have found no difference in patient outcomes when comparing NP and physician-led care in primary care, chronic disease management, or preventive services. Moreover, NP-led care has been associated with higher patient satisfaction, improved access, and lower costs. Bringing this evidence to legislative hearings, policy briefings, and media outlets provides the credibility that policymakers seek. It also counters the safety arguments advanced by opponents, which often lack empirical support. By framing independence as both evidence-based and patient-centered, advocates can shift the debate away from professional turf toward measurable health outcomes.

Public engagement is another essential strategy (American Nurses Association 2021; Nickitas et al. 2020). Advocacy must extend beyond legislative halls to the court of public opinion. Media campaigns, op-eds, social media outreach, and public forums can all be used to raise awareness and build support. Nurses are consistently ranked among the most trusted professionals, and leveraging this trust can help shift public narratives. During the COVID-19 pandemic, when the public saw nurse practitioners on the frontlines, their credibility as autonomous providers grew. Capitalizing on such moments of visibility is vital to sustaining momentum. Digital advocacy, in particular, allows for rapid dissemination of messages and mobilization of supporters. Online petitions, coordinated hashtag campaigns, and storytelling platforms can reach audiences that traditional lobbying cannot.

Cultivating leadership within the NP profession ensures that advocacy efforts are sustainable (Kalb et al. 2022; American Association of Nurse Practitioners 2022). Many NPs are drawn to practice by their commitment to direct patient care, and they may feel unprepared or reluctant to engage in political advocacy. Yet leadership development is critical if the profession is to achieve lasting change. Mentorship programs, advocacy workshops, and opportunities for policy engagement can empower NPs to see themselves not only as clinicians but as leaders. Professional organizations like the American Association of Nurse Practitioners (AANP) play a central role in fostering this leadership, offering resources and training for members to become effective advocates. Nurse practitioner leaders who run for office, serve on health boards, or take executive positions in health organizations further amplify the voice of the profession.

Persistence is perhaps the most important advocacy strategy (Falk-Rafael 2005; Phillips 2022). Legislative victories rarely come quickly. Opponents are well-funded, well-organized, and deeply entrenched in political systems. Advocates must be prepared for setbacks, incremental progress, and long campaigns. The trajectory of NP independence across states illustrates this reality: while some states embraced full practice authority decades ago, others remain resistant despite overwhelming evidence. Advocacy requires patience, resilience, and the ability to adapt strategies as circumstances change. Each legislative session represents an opportunity to advance the conversation, and cumulative efforts gradually erode opposition.

Ultimately, successful advocacy for NP independence must weave together these strategies into a cohesive movement (Nickitas et al. 2020; Mason et al. 2021). Legislative action provides the framework for legal change, coalitions broaden support, evidence provides legitimacy, public engagement builds momentum, leadership sustains progress, and persistence ensures longevity. Together, these elements create a powerful force for transformation, one that not only elevates the role of nurse practitioners but also expands access to care, reduces inequities, and strengthens the US healthcare system.

References

American Association of Nurse Practitioners. Issues at a glance: full practice authority. 2022. https://www.aanp.org.

American Association of Nurse Practitioners. NP fact sheet. 2023. https://www.aanp.org.

American Nurses Association. Code of ethics for nurses with interpretive statements. American Nurses Association; 2015.

American Nurses Association. Nursing advocacy and policy priorities. ANA; 2021. https://www.nursingworld.org.

Buettner-Schmidt K, Lobo ML. Social justice in nursing: a review of the literature. J Adv Nurs. 2012;68(7):1446–57. https://doi.org/10.1111/j.1365-2648.2011.05884.x.

Falk-Rafael AR. (2005). Speaking truth to power: Nursing's legacy and moral imperative. Adv Nurs Sci. 2005;28(3):212–23. https://doi.org/10.1097/00012272-200507000-00005.

Institute of Medicine. The future of nursing: leading change, advancing health. National Academies Press; 2011.

Kalb LG, Stuart EA, Freedman B, Zablotsky B, Vasa RA. Psychiatric-related emergency department visits among children with autism spectrum disorder. J. Autism Dev. Disor. 2022;52(3):997–1008. https://doi.org/10.1007/s10803-021-04917-5.

Kuo YF, Loresto FL, Rounds LR, Goodwin JS. States with the least restrictive regulations experienced the largest increase in patients seen by nurse practitioners. Health Aff. 2013;32(7):1236–43. https://doi.org/10.1377/hlthaff.2013.0072.

Lugo NR, O'Grady ET, Hodnicki D, Hanson CM. Advanced practice registered nurse consensus model report: development and implementation. J Am Acad Nurse Pract. 2007;19(3):141–6. https://doi.org/10.1111/j.1745-7599.2007.00211.x.

Mason DJ, Dickson EL, McLemore MR, Perez GA. Policy & politics in nursing and health care (8th ed.). Elsevier. 2021.

National Academy of Medicine. The future of nursing 2020–2030: charting a path to achieve health equity. National Academies Press; 2021. https://doi.org/10.17226/25982.

National Council of State Boards of Nursing. APRNs in the U.S. NCSBN. 2017. https://www.ncsbn.org.

Nickitas DM, Middaugh D, Aries N. Policy and politics for nurses and other health professionals: Advocacy and action (3rd ed.). Jones & Bartlett Learning. 2020

Phillips SJ. 34th annual legislative update: advancing the APRN movement toward full practice authority. Nurse Pract. 2022;47(1):34–53. https://doi.org/10.1097/01.NPR.0000800186.67836.d4.

Poghosyan L, Liu J, Norful AA, Vonderhaar K. Evaluation of nurse practitioner practice in the United States: a literature review. J Nurse Pract. 2017;13(6):412–22. https://doi.org/10.1016/j.nurpra.2017.01.013.

World Health Organization. State of the world's nursing 2020: investing in education, jobs and leadership. WHO; 2020.

Xue Y, Ye Z, Brewer C, Spetz J. Impact of state nurse practitioner scope-of-practice regulation on health care delivery: systematic review. Nurs Outlook. 2016;64(1):71–85. https://doi.org/10.1016/j.outlook.2015.08.005.

Conclusion

The journey through this book has traced the profound intersections of nursing, social justice, and equity. Each chapter has explored dimensions of inequity, ableism, racial and gender disparities, socioeconomic divides, stigma surrounding mental health, and the struggles faced by LGBTQ+ individuals. What becomes clear is that none of these issues exists in isolation; they overlap, compound, and shape the daily realities of patients and providers alike. The nursing profession, grounded in compassion and advocacy, is uniquely positioned to confront these injustices, not only at the bedside but also in classrooms, boardrooms, legislatures, and communities across the world.

Nursing is more than a set of clinical skills: it is a moral practice, bound by a commitment to human dignity, advocacy, and justice. The themes we have engaged with are not simply abstract ideals; they are lived realities for patients denied access to equitable care, for nurses who encounter discrimination in their own workplaces, and for communities burdened by preventable suffering. To acknowledge inequities is only the first step. The more difficult, and necessary, task is to act to transform recognition into advocacy and advocacy into structural change.

Throughout this book, we have examined how systemic forces such as ableism embedded in healthcare structures, racism perpetuated by inequitable policies, sexism and gender discrimination in the workforce, and the neglect of mental health undermine the principles that nursing strives to uphold. These forces remind us that healthcare is never neutral. It reflects the values, priorities, and power dynamics of the society in which it is situated. Nurses, therefore, cannot afford to be passive participants in this system. They must be active shapers of it, guided by an unwavering commitment to equity.

The call to advocacy is not limited to confronting overt acts of discrimination. It extends to dismantling subtle, normalized practices that perpetuate harm diagnostic overshadowing of disabled patients, implicit bias in treatment decisions, the exclusion of transgender patients from affirming care, or the devaluation of community-based interventions for low-income families. The true measure of nursing's progress toward justice is not how it responds to crises but how it engages with the quiet, everyday injustices that too often remain invisible.

N. Nami, *Unraveling Social Justice Issues in Nursing*,
https://doi.org/10.1007/978-3-032-26512-8

At the same time, this work must be grounded in solidarity. Nurses cannot carry the burden of advocacy alone; change requires partnerships with patients, communities, and interdisciplinary colleagues. It requires humility to listen to those most affected, courage to confront entrenched power structures, and persistence to navigate political and institutional resistance. Solidarity also means recognizing that the struggles for disability rights, racial equity, gender justice, LGBTQ+ inclusion, and mental health parity are interconnected. To advocate for one is to advocate for all, because health equity cannot be achieved piecemeal.

Looking ahead, the future of nursing advocacy will be shaped by global challenges that transcend national borders. Climate change, pandemics, forced migration, and technological transformation will continue to redefine health and healthcare delivery. Nurses will need to expand their vision of advocacy to address not only the inequities in their local communities but also the global structures that shape health. With more than 27 million nurses worldwide, the profession possesses the numbers, credibility, and reach to be a leading voice for planetary health, global solidarity, and justice across borders.

Education will be critical in sustaining this vision. Nursing curricula must embed social justice as a core competency, preparing students to identify inequities and engage in advocacy with the same confidence they bring to clinical care. Faculty and mentors must model advocacy as an integral part of professional identity, not an optional add-on. The next generation of nurses must graduate prepared not only to treat illness but to challenge the systems that produce it.

As this book concludes, its message is simple yet profound: nursing's ethical obligation is inseparable from its social justice mission. To be a nurse is to be an advocate, a change agent, and a defender of human dignity. The future of the profession depends not only on technical expertise but on the willingness to stand against injustice in all its forms.

The work ahead will not be easy. Resistance will persist, setbacks will occur, and progress will be uneven. But nursing's history has always been one of resilience and courage, from Florence Nightingale's reforms in sanitation to the leadership of nurses during the HIV/AIDS crisis and the COVID-19 pandemic. Each generation of nurses has faced its own challenges, and each has risen to meet them. Today's challenge is inequity, and today's nurses must rise to dismantle it.

The vision is clear: a nursing profession that sees advocacy not as an occasional act but as a way of being; a healthcare system that values equity as much as efficiency; and a society in which health is understood as a right, not a privilege. To reach this vision, nurses must continue to speak boldly, act justly, and work collectively. In doing so, they will not only transform healthcare but contribute to building a more compassionate, equitable world for all.

GPSR Compliance

The European Union's (EU) General Product Safety Regulation (GPSR) is a set of rules that requires consumer products to be safe and our obligations to ensure this.

If you have any concerns about our products, you can contact us on ProductSafety@springernature.com

In case Publisher is established outside the EU, the EU authorized representative is:

Springer Nature Customer Service Center GmbH
Europaplatz 3
69115 Heidelberg, Germany

Batch number: 10370712

Printed by Printforce, the Netherlands